# Home Apothecary

*with*

## Ashley English

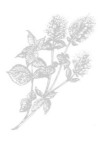

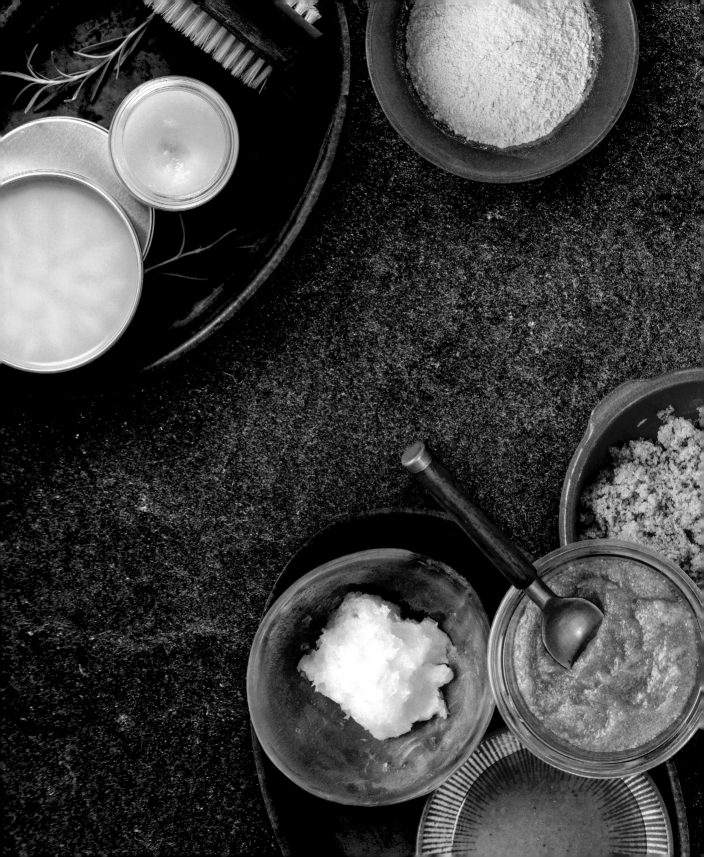

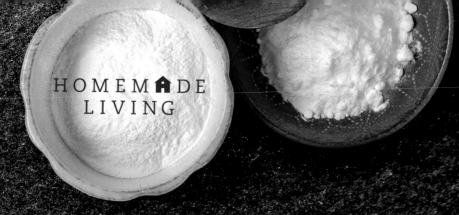

HOMEM🏠DE
LIVING

# Home
# Apothecary

*with*

## Ashley English

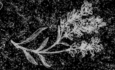

ALL YOU NEED TO KNOW TO CREATE
NATURAL HEALTH AND BODY CARE PRODUCTS

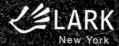

LARK
New York

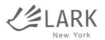

An Imprint of Sterling Publishing Co., Inc.
1166 Avenue of the Americas
New York, NY 10036

ISBN 978-1-4547-1074-5

Distributed in Canada by Sterling Publishing Co., Inc.
c/o Canadian Manda Group, 664 Annette Street
Toronto, Ontario M6S 2C8, Canada
Distributed in the United Kingdom by GMC Distribution Services
Castle Place, 166 High Street, Lewes, East Sussex BN7 1XU, England
Distributed in Australia by NewSouth Books
University of New South Wales, Sydney, NSW 2052, Australia

For information about custom editions, special sales, and premium and corporate purchases, please contact Sterling Special Sales at 800-805-5489 or specialsales@sterlingpublishing.com.

Manufactured in China

2 4 6 8 10 9 7 5 3 1

sterlingpublishing.com
larkcrafts.com

Cover design by David Ter-Avanesyan
Interior design by Shannon Nicole Plunkett
Cover photography by Chris Bain
Interior photography by Erin Adams
Author photo on page 114 by Lynne Harty
Illustrations by iStock/Vladayoung

To Huxley and Alistair, for making me a mama
and allowing me the greatest honor of caring
for the health and wellness of your bodies

# CONTENTS

# Natural Health · 65

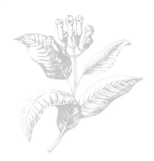

# Introduction

For as long as I can remember, I have loved taking care of others. Caring for other people's physical needs delights me so much that I'm surprised I didn't go into the medical field. When my husband or children get the sniffles, I'm firing up the kettle for hot tea in a dash. When a friend or family member mentions feeling run down or under the weather, I'm quick to recommend a homemade remedy, or, if they're nearby, swing by with a bottle or blend. Creating a home apothecary of handmade health and wellness items is something I began doing when I was in my early twenties and venturing out on my own for the first time. It has since become a passion that has grown and blossomed as I became a wife and a mother.

I've noticed recently that creating a home apothecary has become a growing interest for many others as well. There appears to be a quiet shift taking place. Perhaps you've noticed it too. Not relegated to a specific nation or locale, this gentle transformation won't be found on the streets, but instead at the kitchen table, in the back yard, at the cutting board, and in the medicine cabinet. People ranging from college students to grandparents are making jars of pickles, bottling containers of homebrewed cough syrup, stewarding hives of honeybees, slathering on homemade face masks, and gathering eggs from backyard chickens.

What makes these tasks so profound is that they all involve taking the production of food and health and body care items into your own hands, in the most literal sense. At a time when it's possible to buy any product you want, whenever you want it, from nearly anywhere you shop, the handmade, homegrown, do-it-yourself renaissance advocates for the radical notion that it's okay, and perhaps even necessary, to wait for things, and to take the time to make them yourselves. That nature knows best, and that life truly shines when it's given the opportunity to mature, and age, and ripen to its fullest potential. Essentially, this approach to living is all about slowing down and being mindful of exactly what's going on and into our bodies. No matter what brought you to this book, or whether your interest in all things DIY is limited to creating a home apothecary, welcome to the community of fellow makers and doers! Through bottles of homemade kombucha, jars of lip balm, or loaves of freshly baked sourdough, people around the globe are staking their claim in the realm of what goes into and onto their bodies, for their own vitality, as well as for that of their families, their communities, and this entire shared planet.

I can personally thank Julia Roberts for my introduction to homemade health and wellness products. In the 1991 film *Dying Young*, her character is shown in one scene applying a mayonnaise hair mask. My fifteen-year-old self noted Roberts's luscious locks and decided that I too needed to slather the eggy emulsion onto my own dry tendrils, stat. That inaugural attempt at crafting my own body care product had me hooked.

From there on out, I've been experimenting and tinkering around with building a homemade apothecary. I began playing with homemade face masks next, moving on to teas, cough and cold syrups, and hair rinses from there. At age twenty, I started working retail in natural-foods stores, experimenting in my off-the-clock hours with DIY versions of shelf-ready products. Over the next decade, I spent time everywhere from small, independent mom-and-pop stores to larger, international chains, getting acquainted with all-natural ingredients and tinkering about with homemade remedies. If there's a natural, do-it-yourself alternative to a beauty or health product, I've likely tried to make it at home.

In this book, I share with you the sum collection of all I've learned over several decades of creating a home apothecary. You'll find information on the specific tools you'll need to get started, as well as details on ingredient selection. I've listed the go-to suppliers and distributors I turn to, time after time, for concocting, bottling, and labeling my own apothecary items. Most importantly, the book also contains forty recipes for natural body products and natural health items. When deciding which ones to include in this collection, I sat down with pen and paper and really focused my thinking. I wanted the book to offer those tried-and-true remedies I've been using for years, as well as others that I've incorporated into my health and wellness regimen more recently, when I turned forty and realized that my skin, hair, and insides could benefit from a little more regular TLC and upkeep.

My sincere hope is that this book inspires you deeply. Creating items for my family and loved ones' health and wellness needs has been as rewarding, if not more so, than cooking them a hot breakfast or serving them a nourishing dinner. Knowing that I'm capable of providing myself and others with what our bodies need, whether that's something to soothe a scratchy throat or moisturize dry skin, is empowering beyond description.

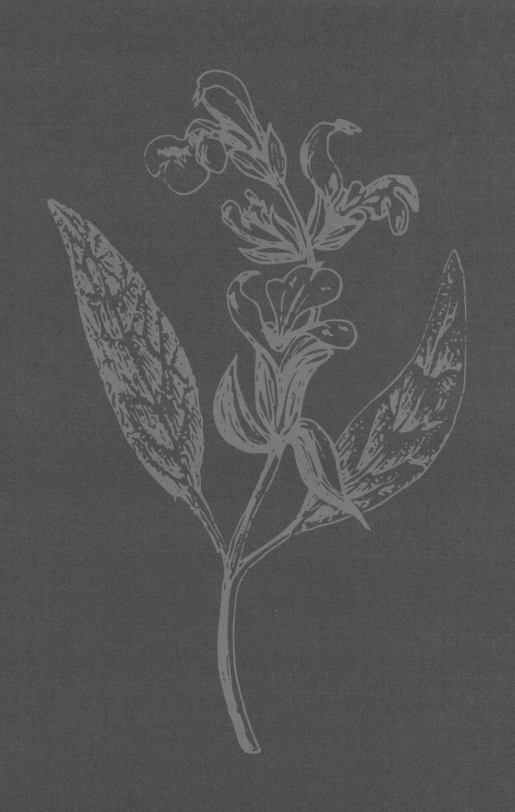

# The Basics

Making homemade remedies for health and wellness can be exceptionally easy. With a few ingredients, some basic pieces of equipment, and a bit of know-how, you're on your way. You don't need a degree in biochemistry or to have completed a medical residency to create homemade mouthwash or a tea for digestion. In this section, I'll introduce you to the ingredients and equipment you'll be working with. This way, you'll be able to gather up the necessary supplies and materials before getting started, as well as know the "why" behind the specific items called for in each recipe. I also share my tried-and-true tips for maintaining the shelf life and integrity of these recipes for as long as possible.

# WHY DIY?

Once upon a time, creating a home apothecary was simply what one did, part of a familiar routine whenever you needed a curative item or product. Aside from the occasional doctor's visit, folk remedies—like sipping peppermint tea for an upset stomach, sprinkling clove powder on an aching tooth, or rubbing tallow on dry skin—were the first solutions that came to mind when you wanted to address your wellness and body care needs. There was no big-box retailer or online boutique to peruse for the ready-made items familiar to us today.

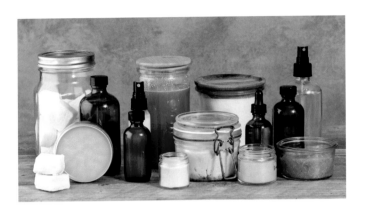

The Industrial Revolution ushered in many changes, including the way home remedies were produced and distributed. Cheap fossil fuels allowed for the advent of refrigeration and long-distance shipping, among other advances. Newly invented preservatives gave chemically manufactured items lengthy shelf lives. And then came the Internet. These days, with one click of a computer mouse or a tap on a smartphone screen, any wellness or body care item under the sun can arrive at your very doorstep, without requiring you to set foot out of the house.

There are, without question, merits to all those technological innovations. That said, there are myriad reasons for crafting a home apothecary of your own. Making your own health and wellness products saves money, eliminates unwanted (and potentially harmful) ingredients, and takes us from the role of the passive consumer, putting us in the driver's seat of producing. In fact, much like in home cooking, the items you'll prepare will be superior in quality and less expensive. Plus, it's just plain fun, which is as good a reason as any to engage in an activity.

Once the required ingredients are procured, you'll be able to craft top-notch, quality items for yourself, your family, and loved ones again and again. Making a jar of scented Bath Salts (page 46) or a bottle of Elderberry & Honey Syrup (page 66) to share with those I love presents a level of care and intimacy that I find deeply rewarding. This is an exciting journey you're embarking on. Here's hoping it affords you the same health and happiness (and cost savings!) it has me.

# INGREDIENTS

One of the best parts of crafting your own health and body care items is that many of the necessary ingredients might already be stored in your pantry, refrigerator, or bathroom cabinets. What you're capable of creating for a home apothecary is well within reach, and at a fraction of the cost of store-bought items of comparable quality and use. Purchasing organic and natural items for home use costs an individual considerably less than they would for larger businesses, who must hire and maintain a staff and place of business, advertise, and then pass those costs on to the consumer. If you think you'll be making home-made items regularly, it might be worth buying ingredients in bulk. Doing so will help reduce your expenses even further.

Familiar items such as baking soda, coconut oil, honey, and milk are just some of the ingredients frequently called for in this book. There will, however, also be items you're perhaps less well acquainted with. Though commonly used in prepared, store-bought health and body care items, they may be wholly foreign if you haven't been dabbling in DIY. Take heart, though. These items, and their benefits and uses, will be covered in this section. Many are commonly found in natural wellness stores, and even some big box retailers. All are readily available online as well. I've listed my go-to online suppliers for these less-common ingredients in the Resources section (page 108).

## ACTIVATED CHARCOAL

This fine black powder is made from charcoal that has been processed at very high temperatures. This results in a product that is more porous than regular charcoal, which helps you to draw out toxins and impurities when taken internally or applied topically.

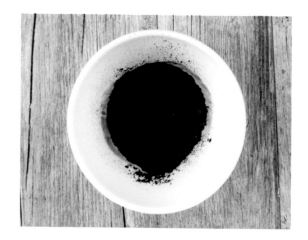

## ALOE VERA GEL

A succulent plant of the genus *aloe*, aloe vera has been cultivated worldwide for agricultural and medicinal uses. The gel inside its leaves

# Organic Certification

Whenever possible (and if your budget allows), I encourage you to use organic ingredients. Organically produced items are free of artificial ingredients and synthetic preservatives. Plus they are grown without the use of toxic pesticides or fertilizers, antibiotics, artificial growth hormones, genetically modified organisms (GMOs), irradiation, and sewage waste.

Rigorous testing and record-keeping is involved in organic certification. In the United States, federally mandated standards require third-party state or private agencies to oversee organic certification for producers. These agencies are, in turn, accredited by the United States Department of Agriculture (USDA). Outside the US, other organizations regulate certification and perform testing to maintain and uphold organic standards globally. While some variation in requirements, regulations, and oversight occurs among countries, they are, by and large, the same internationally.

Why seek out organic ingredients for use of your home apothecary? Anything you ingest or put on your skin affects your overall health and well-being, with health and wellness and body care items being no exception. Organically produced ingredients have been shown to contain greater quantities of nutrients than their conventionally grown counterparts, as well as inherently higher quantities of beneficial fatty acids. Therefore, what you're putting on and in your body will be better for you when organic ingredients are used. Furthermore, organic growing practices are better for the planet. We all live here, so doing what we can to keep this planet verdant and thriving is everyone's responsibility, producers and consumers alike.

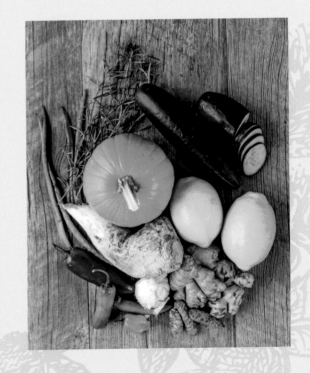

is applied topically for skin problems, such as burns, and ingested to remedy digestive ailments, such as ulcers and heartburn. Aloe vera gel can be purchased at most natural-food stores and even some big-box retailers, as well as online. Alternately, you can keep a plant in your home. Even if you don't need it for sunburns, the plant's gel is helpful should you burn yourself while cooking or baking.

## APPLE CIDER VINEGAR

Created by the fermentation of apples, this type of vinegar is composed of acetic, lactic, citric, and malic acids, as well as enzymes, proteins, and beneficial bacteria. It has a wide range of health and wellness applications and benefits, including controlling blood sugar, improving digestion, and removing dandruff, to name a few.

## ARROWROOT POWDER

Arrowroot powder comes from the rhizomes of several different tropical plants. It's used as a thickener and helps absorb moisture on the skin.

## BAKING SODA

Baking soda is a salt composed of sodium and bicarbonate ions and appears as a fine white powder. It has a wide range of health and wellness applications, from calming skin conditions to whitening teeth and gently exfoliating skin.

## BEESWAX

Beeswax, which is secreted by honeybees when they construct honeycombs, contains antibacterial properties and has the ability to soften and thicken health and wellness products. It also hydrates and protects skin.

## BUTTERS

Botanically derived butters have numerous benefits to the skin. Shea, cocoa, and mango butters hydrate and nourish deeply.

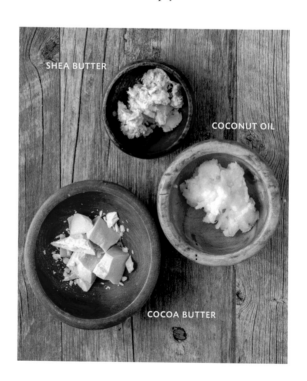

SHEA BUTTER

COCONUT OIL

COCOA BUTTER

**COCOA BUTTER:** Derived from cocoa beans, this butter smells just like chocolate! It's full of fats that help to nourish and moisturize skin.

**MANGO BUTTER:** Sourced from cold-pressing mango seeds, this butter, as with cocoa and shea butters, moisturizes without feeling greasy.

**SHEA BUTTER:** Extracted from the nut of the African shea tree, this butter can deeply nourish dry skin.

## CALCIUM POWDER

Used for the Healthy Mouth Tooth Powder (page 98), calcium powder strengthens and whitens teeth by polishing tooth enamel and removing stains. Look for the calcium carbonate form when purchasing.

## CARRIER OILS

Sourced from nuts or seeds, these plant-based oils are most typically used for diluting essential oils, to help safely "carry" them onto the skin for use. They also offer moisturizing, healing, protecting, and soothing properties. Most are entirely or nearly odorless. Some examples include apricot kernel oil, argan oil, coconut oil, grapeseed oil, jojoba oil, olive oil, rosehip seed oil, safflower oil, sesame oil, and sweet almond oil. I call for several different carrier oils in this book and specify which one to use in each project's ingredients listing.

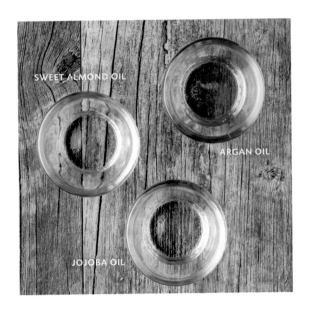

## CITRIC ACID

Citric acid is a crystalline acid naturally occurring in sour fruits, including citrus. It is produced for commercial use by fermenting sugar and used here to make the Bath Fizzies (page 52) bubble. You can purchase it in a powdered, granular form.

## CLAYS

Cosmetic clays have a wide range of skin care uses, providing nourishment and drawing out and cleansing impurities that are both on the surface and embedded within.

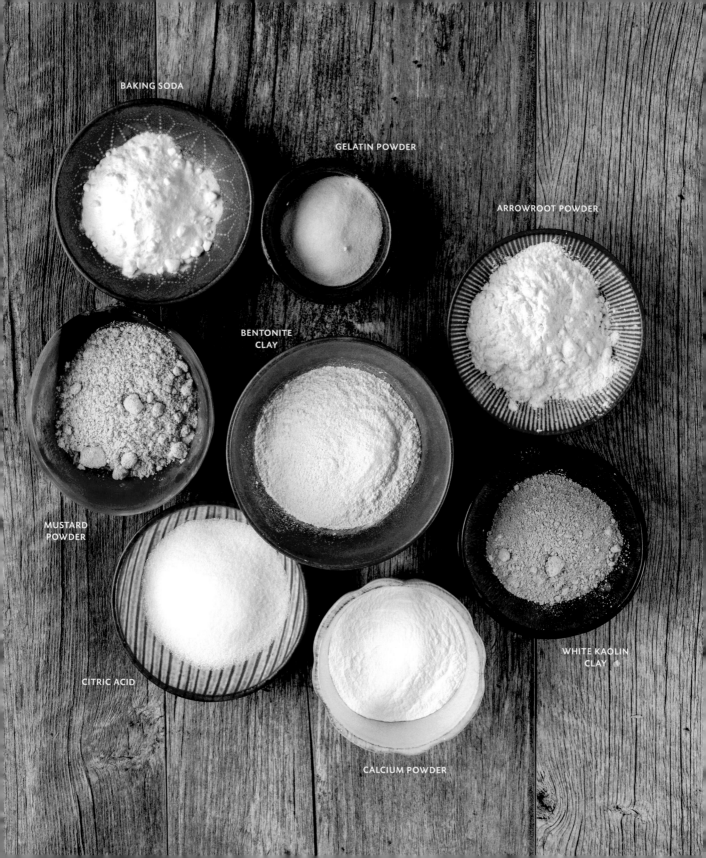

BAKING SODA

GELATIN POWDER

ARROWROOT POWDER

BENTONITE
CLAY

MUSTARD
POWDER

WHITE KAOLIN
CLAY

CITRIC ACID

CALCIUM POWDER

BENTONITE CLAY: Derived from volcanic ash, this clay is named after Fort Benton, Montana, and the Benton Shale, so named by geologist Wilbur C. Knight in 1898. These days, bentonite clay is used to describe any number of absorbent clays, even though they might be sourced from other locations. They assist with digestion, improve skin health, and remove toxins, among other uses.

WHITE KAOLIN CLAY: A fine, light powder, this clay is used in a wide range of cosmetic and body care applications. It is considered the gentlest of all clays; it helps activate circulation in the skin and also exfoliates and cleanses it.

## DISTILLED WATER

Distilled water has been boiled into vapor and then condensed back into liquid in a different container. Any impurities in the original water are removed, leaving behind a purified water. It is used extensively in cosmetics and wellness products as a deterrent to bacterial growth.

## DAIRY

In this book, milk and yogurt are included in several remedies. I used whole-fat versions of both when creating the recipes that feature these ingredients. Lactic acid, a type of alpha hydroxy acid found in dairy, helps penetrate and loosen up the uppermost layers of skin cells, resulting in a natural shedding process. As dead cells slough off, newly formed skin cells rise to the surface, with the end result reducing visible signs of aging. Furthermore, dairy products contain vitamins, minerals, enzymes, fats, and proteins that benefit the skin. If at all possible, opt for organic dairy.

## EPSOM SALTS

Epsom salts is the common name of the inorganic salt magnesium sulfate. It is used to soothe sore muscles, support stress reduction, reduce pain and swelling, and improve skin tone and circulation.

## ESSENTIAL OILS

Essential oils are concentrated aromatic extracts derived from a wide range of botanicals, including seeds, roots, flowers, bark, and stems. Essential oils are regularly employed in the home apothecary. They are extracted from the botanicals by the processes of distillation and cold-pressing, and typically require a good deal of plant matter to produce just a small amount of product, which accounts for their high cost. That said, owing to the intense concentration of aromatic compounds in a single drop, essential oils go far. A small bottle should last quite some time.

# Essential Oils: Benefits & Uses

Essential oils are valuable ingredients to include in a home apothecary. I turn to my collection nearly every day for a wide range of applications. Aside from just smelling good, these concentrated oils offer numerous therapeutic uses. Here are some of the properties of the oils called for in this book.

**CLARY SAGE:** Helpful for circulation and hormone balancing.

**CEDAR:** Relaxing to the mind and body, as well as a great pest deterrent.

**CHAMOMILE:** Helpful for insomnia, calming to the mind, beneficial for skin health.

**CLOVE:** Antibacterial, helpful for tooth pain, mildly analgesic.

**CORIANDER:** Helpful for detoxification and digestion.

**EUCALYPTUS:** Addresses respiratory issues, including congestion, cough, bronchitis, and allergies.

**FIR:** Helpful for aches and pains, as well as respiratory concerns.

**FRANKINCENSE:** Acts as an anti-inflammatory, immunity booster, and mood balancer.

**GERANIUM:** Uplifting for mood, as well as cleansing and detoxification. Aids with dry skin and wrinkles.

**GRAPEFRUIT:** Helpful with stress management, as well as weight concerns.

**LAVENDER:** Calming, helpful for skin concerns, including burns, bites, and wounds.

**LEMONGRASS:** Supports the lymphatic system, uplifting and invigorating for mood.

**LIME:** Elevates mood, helps increase focus and concentration.

**PEPPERMINT:** Helpful for head tension and headaches, digestion, and alertness.

**ROSEMARY:** Aids in mental fatigue and focus, bolsters immunity.

**SANDALWOOD:** A mood elevator, helps with concentration.

**SPRUCE:** Helpful for respiratory concerns and viral infections.

**TANGERINE:** Uplifting, as well as immune-boosting.

**TEA TREE:** Detoxifies and cleanses and has antibacterial, antiviral, and antifungal properties.

**WINTERGREEN:** Anti-inflammatory, mood-boosting, and is helpful for aches and pains.

**YLANG-YLANG:** Elevates mood, balances hormones, and is helpful for elevated blood pressure and restlessness.

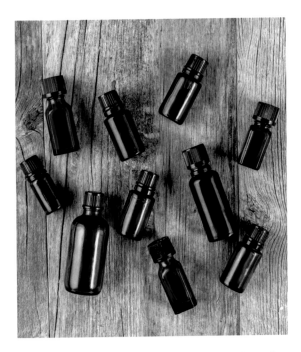

The compounds giving these oils their fragrances are highly volatile, meaning they'll quickly evaporate and lose their potency and efficacy if directly exposed to oxygen. Store them with their lids on when not in use, and place the containers in a cool location, away from direct sunlight or high heat.

Take great care when using these products. Applying them directly to the skin can be quite painful, so always use a carrier oil for dilution. I speak from experience here, as I once severely burned my skin after getting into a bath filled with hot water and multiple undiluted drops of grapefruit essential oil. Keep essential oils away from the eye area, as well as away from the lips, mouth, and nasal passages. Several essential oils can increase photosensitivity to the sun, especially citrus-derived oils such as lime, orange, lemon, grapefruit, and bergamot. It's best to avoid direct sun exposure for several hours after using these particular oils. As with all products, natural or otherwise, keep them out of the reach of children, and consult your physician before use if you're pregnant.

A wide range of essential oils is available for purchase. It can be difficult to know which are reputable and carry pure, unadulterated compounds, and which are mixed with synthetics. In general, avoid any item with wording such as "perfume" or "fragrance" oil, as these are synthetically derived and are not pure plant extracts. I've listed several of my favorite essential oil companies, a number of which I have used for decades with great results, in the Resources section (page 108).

## GELATIN POWDER

Gelatin is derived from the collagen found in animal skin, bones, and connective tissue after they break down. We'll be using powdered gelatin here, which is produced by first drying the gelatin, and then breaking it up into tiny grains. Vegetarians and vegans can seek out powdered agar (sometimes called agar-agar) as a replacement.

Agar is made from a type of algae and can be used interchangeably with the gelatin.

## HERBS & SPICES

A number of recipes in this book call for herbs or spices. While many, such as fresh rosemary, will be familiar to you, others, such as elderberry or calendula, may be less so. If you have a natural-food store in your area, they likely have a bulk herbs and spices area, which is where I'd recommend sourcing your ingredients from. That way, you can purchase only the amount needed to make whatever it is you're creating, thereby keeping your herbs and spices as fresh as possible. Of course, if you intend to make a large batch at once, perhaps for gifting purposes or simply because you know your household will go through something pretty quickly, then I suggest purchasing a larger bulk amount. For such needs, I recommend seeking an online supplier (see Resources section on page 108). Store any unused herbs or spices in either a paper bag secured with a clip or rubber band, or, best of all, in a lidded glass container. Either way, keep your herbs and spices in a cool, dry area, away from direct heat.

It has long been a dream of mine to source all, or at least most, of the botanical ingredients used in my home apothecary remedies from my own yard. While I'm still well on my way to realizing that end goal, I have a number of plants established in my medicinal garden. If you have the space, time, and inclination, I invite you to consider growing plants of your own. For drying herbs, I suggest bundling bunches together and hanging them upside down indoors until they are fully dried. Store the dried herbs in a lidded glass container, and place it in a cool, dry location out of direct sunlight. Alternately, use a multi-shelf food dehydrator if you have one on hand or if you plan on growing (and drying) a large quantity of herbs at a time.

## LIQUOR

Several remedies here call for spirits such as vodka, tequila, and grain alcohol. Organic versions are ideal; but, if unavailable, conventional versions are completely fine to use.

## LIQUID STEVIA

Stevia is a sweetener sourced from the leaves of the plant *Stevia rebaudiana* and considered a sugar substitute. It's also available in powdered form.

## MILK OF MAGNESIA

Milk of magnesia is a white suspension of hydrated magnesium carbonate in water. In this book, it is used as a natural deodorant.

# Herbs & Spices: Benefits & Uses

I call for a number of herbs and spices in their whole or fresh form here. Each has long been heralded for various therapeutic applications. Here are some of those uses.

**CALENDULA:** Helpful for swelling, pain, and inflammation, as well as wound-healing and dry skin.

**CINNAMON:** Antibacterial, antiviral, and anti-inflammatory; helpful for balancing blood pressure and blood sugar.

**CHAMOMILE:** Antiseptic and anti-inflammatory; helpful for a range of skin conditions.

**CHILI PEPPERS:** The heat from chilis moves phlegm out of the throat and sinuses. Peppers are also a wonderful source of vitamin C, which is helpful for bolstering immunity.

**CLOVES:** Anti-inflammatory and antibacterial; helps with tooth pain and freshens breath.

**ELDERBERRIES:** Antiviral and high in antioxidants, making it helpful for cold and flu treatment and prevention.

**FENNEL SEEDS:** Helpful for digestive and respiratory concerns.

**GINGER:** Aids in digestion and the management of blood sugar and cholesterol levels.

**HORSERADISH:** Antibacterial; promotes blood flow, and helpful for fighting the common cold.

**MUSTARD POWDER:** Helpful for aches and pains, as well as respiratory congestion.

**ROSEMARY:** Improves blood circulation and helps in reducing stress and anxiety.

**PEPPERMINT:** Addresses digestive concerns and helps with headaches and cold and flu prevention.

**SAGE:** Anti-inflammatory, aids with skin and digestive concerns.

**SLIPPERY ELM BARK:** Useful for sore throats, as it leaves a mucilaginous (or slimy) coating; also helpful for digestive concerns and wound healing.

**SPEARMINT:** Anti-inflammatory and helpful for digestive concerns, headaches, and oral care issues.

**TARRAGON:** Antibacterial; helpful with digestive concerns, and beneficial to the nervous system.

**TURMERIC:** Anti-inflammatory, helpful with cardiovascular health and managing cholesterol and stress levels.

**WILD CHERRY BARK:** Addresses a range of respiratory issues and digestive concerns, and assists with pain management.

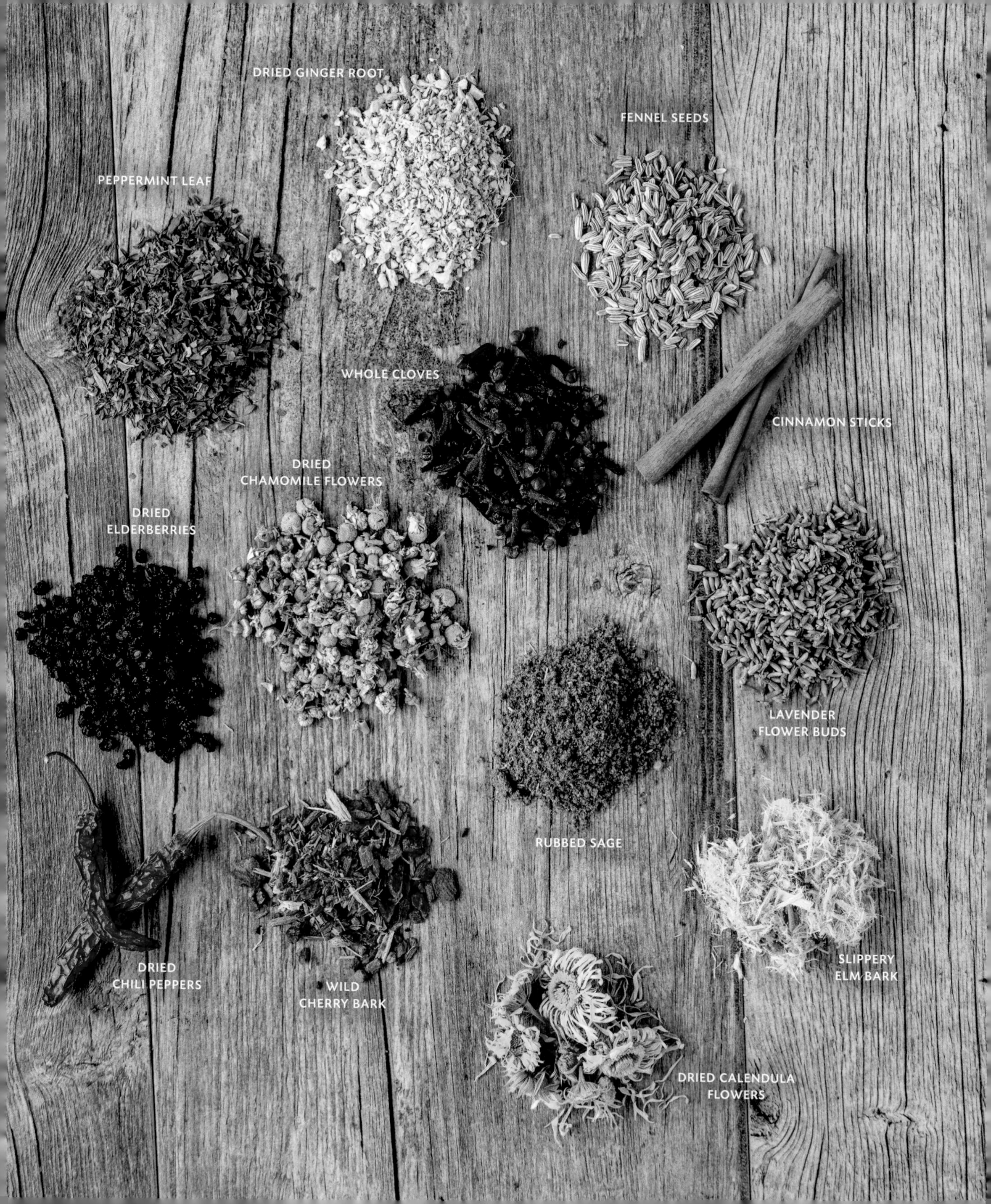

DRIED GINGER ROOT

FENNEL SEEDS

PEPPERMINT LEAF

WHOLE CLOVES

CINNAMON STICKS

DRIED
CHAMOMILE FLOWERS

DRIED
ELDERBERRIES

LAVENDER
FLOWER BUDS

RUBBED SAGE

DRIED
CHILI PEPPERS

WILD
CHERRY BARK

SLIPPERY
ELM BARK

DRIED CALENDULA
FLOWERS

## NATURAL COLORING & FLAVORING

Very few recipes in this book call for colorings or flavorings. For those that do, though, I suggest naturally sourced versions, such as plant-derived colorings and flavorings like peppermint and orange extract. Keep artificial colorings and flavorings, or any artificial ingredients, out of your home apothecary to avoid unintentionally exposing family or friends to ingredients that might make them ill. My oldest son is highly allergic to artificial food dyes. (We learned this the hard way when the dentist accidentally gave him a lollipop containing artificial food coloring.)

## RAW HONEY

A sweet liquid food produced by honeybees, honey is used in health and wellness applications internally and topically. It helps the skin pull in and retain moisture and is antibacterial and anti-microbial. As for internal benefits, honey is packed with nutrients and antioxidants, making it beneficial to the immune system. Raw honey is honey which has not been heat-treated in any way, and will be indicated as such on its packaging.

## ROSEWATER

Obtained by steam distillation of rose petals, this scented water is imbued with tiny droplets of rose essential oil given off in the distillation process. Rosewater is used in both cosmetics and food. Used topically, it can help reduce redness, heal minor skin injuries, and remedy infections.

## WITCH HAZEL

Created by steaming twigs of the witch hazel plant, witch hazel is anti-inflammatory and anti-microbial. It helps tighten and clean pores, as well as cool and soothe irritated skin.

## XYLITOL POWDER

Xylitol is a sugar alcohol that is used as a sugar substitute because its chemical structure stimulates taste receptors for sweetness on the tongue. It's found in tiny amounts in a number of fruits and vegetables regularly consumed in most people's diets, from corn to berries. In this book, xylitol is used in my Healthy Mouth Tooth Powder (page 98).

# EQUIPMENT

As with your ingredients, the equipment needed for your home apothecary consists of tools that you might already have in your kitchen. Your kitchen can do double duty as both the place to whip up nutritious, creative meals and the nucleus of your home remedy crafting.

I'm a big fan of appropriating things for new and (potentially) unconventional uses. I love this form of "upcycling," as it allows me to repurpose items within reach without the need to spend, or for new objects to be manufactured. Look around your kitchen and assess what you might have on hand.

Anything missing? Time to hit up the thrift and secondhand shops! You'll likely be able to source many of the items that you'll need to create home apothecary items from such places. You can purchase anything that remains on your list online (see Resources, page 108).

## BLENDER or FOOD PROCESSOR

For several recipes, you'll need a blender or food processor to fully incorporate all the ingredients. A machine dedicated to crafting home apothecary products is ideal to have around. The scent of some products, such as essential oils, and the texture of others, like beeswax, can linger even after cleaning, so reserving a blender or food processor exclusively for such projects is especially handy. That said, don't feel as though it's absolutely essential to run out and purchase or procure a machine expressly for home apothecary projects. The scent and

materials left on food processor or blender basins will eventually go away after several washings, especially if you run them through a hot dishwasher.

## BOTTLES, JARS & CONTAINERS

Just about every project you'll make in this book will need to be stored somewhere, aside from those intended to be used up entirely in one sitting. That's where having a variety of jars on hand comes into play. From upcycled and repurposed glass bottles to newly purchased mason jars, there's certainly no shortage of options, as long as the container is safe for holding foodstuff. If you intend to gift any of these items, you can easily find a wide array of attractive glass bottles and jars at craft stores, big-box retailers, and online.

For the most part, I prefer to use glass or metal containers in my home apothecary. That's a personal, as well as aesthetic, preference, but it also comes in part from the propensity of certain ingredients like essential oils to leave lingering aromas and to degrade plastic over time. However, for several remedies, including High & Dry Baby Powder (page 59), Apple Cider Vinegar Rinse (page 27), and Germ-Busting Hand Sanitizer (page 89), I do use plastic containers expressly dedicated to those specific products. The choice to use plastic or not for other remedies is entirely up to you.

Tinted, dark blue, or amber-colored glass bottles are especially helpful for some body care projects, such as the Everyday Face Oil (page 35) and Baby Massage Oil (page 62). These contain oils (including essential oils) that are rendered less effective if exposed to the heat generated by sunlight. Metal tins or bottles are another option, especially for items such as salves or lip balm.

Most of the remedies use standard screw-on lids, but several call for specialized caps, including droppers and spray nozzles or misters. For these kinds of toppers, you can opt to upcycle, using lids from purchased products whose contents have been used, or purchasing new ones. Upcycling is my typical go-to.

## CANDY THERMOMETER

A candy thermometer, which is a large, tubular thermometer with a metal clip that allows you to attach it to the side of a pot, will be necessary to make the Soothing Spiced Cough Drops (page 80). These types of thermometers allow you to observe both the temperature and the stage of a sugar solution. These stages, such as the hard crack stage, determine how the finished product will turn out and are crucial to keep track of during the cooking process. While there are a number of techniques and tricks for determining the temperature and stage of a sugar solution without the help of a thermometer, having one on hand removes the guesswork.

Candy thermometers are available both in the more traditional liquid format that consists of a glass tube, and in digital form. Digital candy thermometers tend to gauge temperature more quickly and accurately, and some also have settings that alert you when a target temperature has been reached. You can source both formats easily from kitchen supply stores or online.

## DOUBLE BOILER

A double boiler, also known as a *bain marie*, uses steam to melt, cook, or warm a food item. It consists of two components, a large pot filled with hot or boiling water, and a smaller pot that fits inside the larger one. The smaller pot uses the steam from the water in the larger pot to process the food. The heat is provided indirectly, making it ideal for gently melting or warming up ingredients.

## FINE-MESH SIEVE

A fine-mesh sieve is an indispensable tool in one's home apothecary for straining herbs in products like the Elderberry & Honey Syrup

# DIY Double Boiler

If you do not have a double boiler, it's very easy to fashion a DIY version:

1. Begin by placing several inches of water in the bottom of a pot.

2. Place a heat-proof mixing bowl on top of the pot. The bowl shouldn't be in direct contact with the water, so be sure to use one that can rest above liquid in the pot below. There should be space between the mixing bowl and the water.

3. Bring the water to a simmer. Place the required ingredients in the mixing bowl, and proceed with the project's instructions.

(page 66) or Rosemary Hair Oil (page 28). Sieves come in a wide range of sizes; I'd opt for one that is about 5 to 9 inches (12.7 to 22.9 cm) in diameter. A sieve dedicated for home apothecary use would be lovely, but it's also perfectly fine to employ the same sieve for home cooking as long as you wash it thoroughly in between uses with a dishwasher or hot, soapy water.

## FUNNEL

It's useful to have funnels in a range of sizes for bottling purposes. Whether you opt for plastic or metal is entirely up to you. Do keep in mind, however, that projects using essential oils tend to leave a fragrance behind on plastic. Plastic also breaks down more quickly over time.

## LABELS

If there's one tip I hope to stress above all others in this book, it's to label, label, label. The last thing you want is to mistake your Decongestant Balm (page 78) for your Lip Balm (page 44), all because you forgot to label them. Similarly, while the Elderberry & Honey Syrup (page 66) is delicious, you wouldn't want to mistake it in the refrigerator for a bottle of blackberry syrup and pour it all over a stack of hot pancakes. I speak from experience here. Learn from my mistakes, and label every product you create, whether you're storing them in the medicine cabinet, on the bathroom shelves, or in the refrigerator.

Dating your remedies is also especially helpful, as certain items have a shorter shelf life than others. You'll want to note both when it was made, and its expiration date. A massive array of labels is readily available for purchase, from craft stores, to office supply stores, to websites like Etsy. You can use blank labels and hand-write the information about your bottle or jar's contents, or use a home printer for more uniform, consistent lettering or to experiment with a variety of fonts. You can also use paper tags, tying them onto the containers with twine or string, and reuse them until they wear out. Just remember to cross out and update the made/use-by dates each time.

## MEASURING CUPS & SPOONS

You'll use measuring cups and spoons more than any other tool in your home apothecary tool kit, so invest in a well-made set. In my own tool kit, I use both metal measuring cups and spoons and glass measuring cups. Heatproof glass measuring cups with pourable spouts and handles are incredibly helpful when you're measuring and pouring liquids. They also come in a range of sizes, from those measuring ¼–1 cup (60–240 ml), to those with 2-cup (480 ml), 4-cup (360 ml), and 8-cup (720 ml) volumes.

Make your selection based on the overall quantity of projects you'll be making. While you might be primarily making items for only your and your family's needs, you might want to double, triple, or quadruple the amounts called for in some recipes for other occasions, such as for holiday gift-giving purposes. Larger-

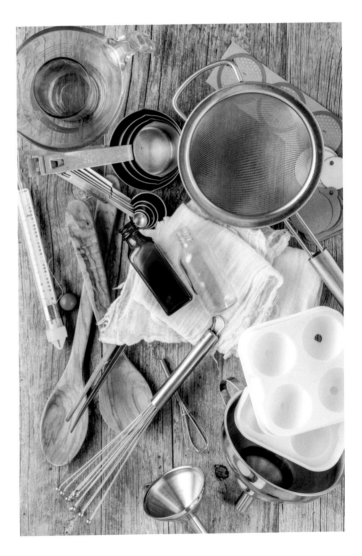

capacity glass measuring cups work well during those times.

## MIXING BOWLS

When you mix up your creations, you'll need somewhere to contain them. Bowls are ever present in my home apothecary tool kit — and, well, let's just say that the collection in my home is *abundant* and leave it at that. While you certainly don't need to assemble a bowl collection anywhere close to the scale of mine, you will want to have at least a few options on hand in a range of sizes. I recommend glass, ceramic, and metal bowls. Plastic bowls are best avoided in the home apothecary tool kit, as they tend to hold on to fragrances and colors (such as with essential oils or turmeric and charcoal). You'll also want to be sure to include at least a few heatproof bowls, especially if you'll be making a DIY double boiler (page 17). It might be worth keeping a dedicated bowl for those projects that use beeswax, as removing the wax can be a colossal task, especially if it has hardened.

## MUSLIN or CHEESECLOTH

For certain projects, no sieve is quite fine enough to thoroughly strain your liquids. That's where unbleached muslin (sometimes referred to as "butter muslin") and cheesecloth can help.

Muslin is a tightly woven natural cloth that can catch those minute particles that might otherwise slip through a sieve's openings. Cheesecloth works similarly, as long as you use a variety with a tight, close weave. Avoid the loosely woven, flimsier versions typically found in grocery stores. Muslin can be found at fabric stores or online. Whatever you choose, I suggest giving it a quick, gentle wash in cold water and drying it thoroughly before the first use. Both materials are reusable, as long as they are washed and dried completely between uses.

## SILICONE MOLDS

For Bath Fizzies (page 52), you'll need to have a set of silicone molds on hand. The recipe makes around a dozen ¼-cup (60 ml) fizzies, so seek out a mold containing that number of slots, or purchase several molds with fewer spaces. Silicone molds are available in a wide array of styles and shapes. From holiday motifs to geometric shapes, there's one for every inclination and occasion.

## STIRRING UTENSILS

When bentonite clay comes into contact with metal, its effectiveness is reduced considerably. That's why some products, such as with the Tooth Powder (page 98) or Diaper Cream (page

60), specifically call for a wooden chopstick or spoon for stirring. Otherwise, most of the remedies in this book require stirring of some form or another, and a whisk or metal spoon will work perfectly fine if a wooden chopstick or spoon isn't specifically mentioned.

## SAFETY GUIDELINES

As with any DIY item, whether made in a sterilized lab or a home kitchen, an ounce of prevention is worth a pound of cure. It's a huge bummer to have invested time and money in creating a home remedy, only for it to go awry. To that end, here are several precautions to help you keep your lovingly crafted items in their best possible condition.

### STERILIZING CONTAINERS

Whatever vessels you end up choosing for your finished items, it's essential that they be as clean as possible to prevent contamination and spoilage. This is best achieved by sterilization.

To sterilize jars and bottles, you have several options. They can be run through a dishwasher, boiled in hot water for 10 minutes, or heated in

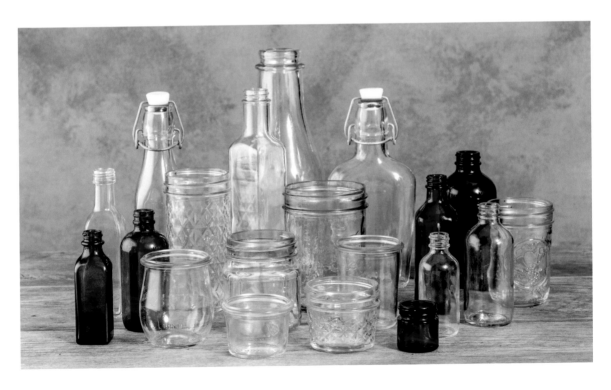

a 275°F (135°C) oven for 20 minutes (the oven method works for glass and metal containers, but not for any plastic items). No matter which route you select, always sterilize your containers on the same day, or the night before, that you intend to fill them (as opposed to several days prior). Furthermore, make sure each one is completely dry before filling. You don't want any lingering moisture to contaminate your finished product. This is best achieved by either sterilizing and drying your containers in the dishwasher or oven first thing in the morning, or, if you're using the boiling-water method, doing so the night before you plan to make your remedies, and leaving them to dry overnight. As for sterilizing lids, they can be processed in the same manner as jars and bottles, but avoid putting any plastic lids into the oven.

When you have finished the contents of a container, use a bottle brush to remove any remaining residue. Then either place the containers upside down in the dishwasher and wash on a normal setting, or use hot soapy water and wash by hand. Dry thoroughly before storing.

## SHELF LIFE

Each item in this book has a recommended shelf life. Take care to follow that recommendation closely. You can make this easy for yourself by labeling your items with the date they were made and the date they should be used by. Follow the storage recommendations, whether they advise you to keep your products in the refrigerator, in a cool location, or away from the sun.

## AVOID BACTERIAL & FUNGAL GROWTH

You can easily avoid bacterial and fungal growth by keeping your finished item away from your mouth and by avoiding exposure to something that has been in your mouth. For example, don't take a spoonful of Hot Honey (page 72), put the spoon in your mouth, and then dip the same spoon back into the same honey jar for another spoonful. If a product calls for distilled water, make sure to use it. This will extend shelf life and prevent bacterial growth on and in your remedies. The adage with foodstuffs, "when in doubt, throw it out," applies here as well. If you suspect that an item is "off," owing to visible or olfactory cues (in other words, it looks or smells gross), trust your gut and toss it.

## USE FRESH INGREDIENTS

Fresh is always best. Though it might seem frugal to use the bag of dried spearmint that you purchased two years ago and just found crumpled in the corner of your pantry, put it in the compost. You might not be able to see mold or mildew on old ingredients. Plus, these items lose efficacy over time. As with your finished products, label and date any herbs or spices you purchase in bulk, and aim to use them within 9 to 12 months. I always recommend an annual pantry purge. I use the days around the new year for the task.

## ADVERSE REACTIONS (AND WHAT TO DO)

If you should have a negative reaction to any remedy here, immediately discontinue using it and dispose of the remaining contents so that others won't also become ill. Negative reactions include difficulty breathing, severe nausea,

vomiting, profuse diarrhea, skin reactions, hives, or any other type of reaction that appears to directly follow use of a remedy. If you suspect poisoning, or your pet or child consumes a large amount of any product, call Poison Control at 1-800-222-1222. Always keep your home apothecary items out of the reach of pets and children, as with any wellness and body care items, whether store-bought or homemade.

## CONSULT A MEDICAL PROFESSIONAL

To rule out possible contraindications, those who are breast-feeding or pregnant, taking prescription medications, are very young or very old, or are otherwise immune-compromised should consult their physicians before administering any recipe contained in this book.

# A Note on Preservatives

Aside from vitamin E, I've opted to avoid the use of preservatives in this book. This is due in part to the fact that, for me, these remedies are natural products, much in the same manner as foods. As such, they have a relatively short shelf life, and need to be consumed or used up in a timely manner (as indicated in each recipe's notes). Additionally, preservatives can be costly, so I elected to avoid them altogether here.

# Gift-Giving Packages

A number of the remedies in this book would make wonderful gifts, especially when thoughtfully bundled with a few other similarly themed items. As for what to put the items in, wicker baskets make great gifting receptacles. I keep a stash on hand at all times expressly for this purpose, since I've found baskets very easy to source at great prices, especially at secondhand stores. Here are several suggestions for gifting concepts.

**Treat Yourself**

A lovely gift combination for someone in desperate need of relaxation would be a bottle of Bath Oil (page 49) and a jar of Blissful Bath Salts (page 46), perhaps tucked into a basket with a box of tea or bottle of wine, a chocolate bar, and a loofah or skin brush.

**Baby Love**

If you know some soon-to-be parents, a gift trio of Baby Massage Oil (page 62), a bottle of High & Dry Baby Powder (page 59), and a container of Bottoms Up Diaper Cream (page 60) would make a lovely present, perhaps coupled with a receiving blanket and a burping cloth.

**Catch Some Zzz's**

Anyone going through a particularly challenging time, whether owing to a new baby or a stressful situation such as a move or divorce, would benefit from this package. Alongside a container of Sleep Salve (page 90), include an eye pillow and a packet of bedtime tea.

# Natural Body

Tending to our external bodies is just as vital as tending to their inner bits. From hair to skin and hands, it all needs tender, loving care, offered regularly and routinely. However, the cost of many shelf-ready body care items is often prohibitively expensive—and they frequently contain chemicals that are best avoided. That's why I love turning my do-it-yourself tendency on, well, myself! Crafting body care products at home saves considerable money and allows me to experiment and play with fragrances and remedies specific to my body's needs, as well as those of my family. Furthermore, it's always a real treat to gift a loved one or friend with a self-care product you've made expressly with them in mind. Doing so nourishes body *and* soul.

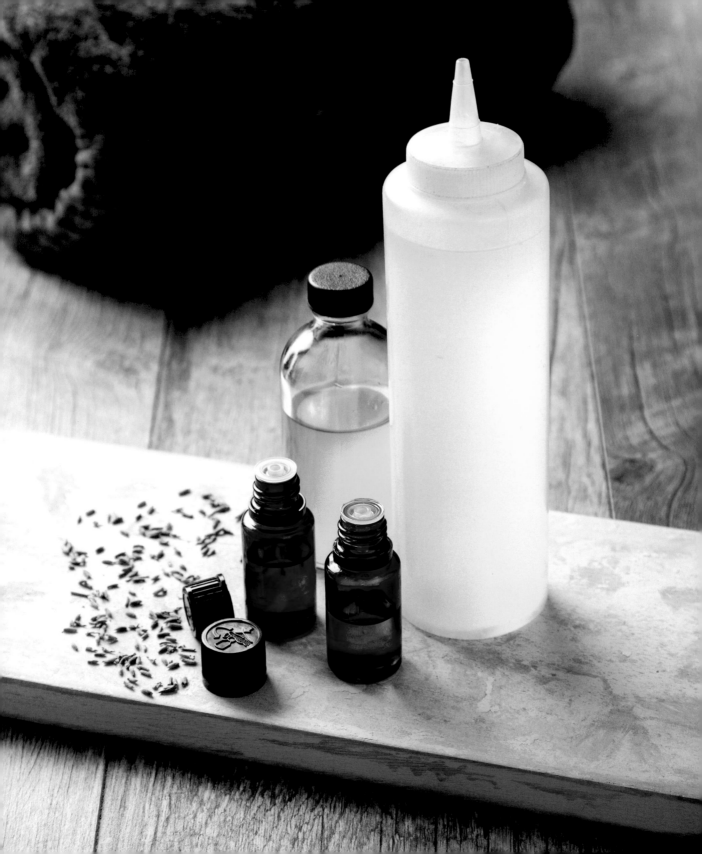

# APPLE CIDER VINEGAR RINSE

I've experienced dry scalp nearly my entire adulthood. I've tried nearly every natural remedy for this problem, from medicated shampoos to moisturizing masks. It wasn't until I began applying this home-made apple cider vinegar rinse that the flakiness I've battled for decades began to disappear. Apple cider vinegar has acetic acid, which helps restore and balance the scalp's pH level and keep moisture in place. A properly balanced scalp pH results in shiny, lustrous, properly nourished hair. Lavender and tea tree essential oils not only provide a lovely fragrance but also combat dandruff and soothe irritated skin.

**Yield:** 1 application • **Frequency of use:** Use once a week. • **Storage:** Do not store. Use immediately.

## » To Prepare:

1. Combine all the ingredients in a plastic squeeze bottle. Secure the cap on the bottle and shake vigorously to fully mix all ingredients together.

2. To use, hop into the shower and shampoo your hair as normal. After rinsing the shampoo out, lean your head forward and squirt the entire contents of the bottle directly onto your scalp, taking care to avoid the eye area. Leave on for at least 1 minute, and up to 4 minutes.

3. Rinse thoroughly with warm water. Shampooing again isn't necessary, as the vinegar odor will fade as your hair dries. If you regularly use conditioner after shampooing, go ahead and apply it now.

4. Towel your hair dry, then allow it to fully air-dry.

## » You Will Need:

¼ cup (60 ml) apple cider vinegar

1½ cups (355 ml) warm water*

2 drops lavender essential oil

2 drops tea tree essential oil

One 16-ounce (480 ml) plastic squeeze bottle

* *Using warm, not hot, water will ensure a more pleasant experience when you pour the solution onto your scalp.*

# ROSEMARY HAIR OIL

I turn to this hair oil treatment, along with the Apple Cider Vinegar Rinse (page 27), to keep my scalp nourished and my hair shiny, smooth, and free from split ends. Rosemary can increase scalp circulation, which in turn facilitates hair growth and alleviates a dry or itchy scalp. Lavender calms irritated skin. Do like I do and choose a quiet evening at home, slip on your comfiest pj's, apply the oil, and put on a riveting movie or curl up with a spellbinding read, while the oil works its magic.

Yield: 1 cup (240 ml), approximately four applications • Frequency of use: Use once every two weeks (about twice monthly). • Storage: Store in a cool, dark area. Use within 6 months.

## » You Will Need:

1 cup (240 ml) sweet almond oil or apricot kernel oil

5 sprigs fresh rosemary

5 drops rosemary essential oil

5 drops lavender essential oil

One 8-ounce (240 ml) bottle

## » To Prepare:

1. In a double boiler or a DIY version (see page 17 for instructions), combine the almond oil and rosemary sprigs.

2. Bring the water in the double boiler or pot to a gentle simmer, then reduce heat to the lowest setting and leave to simmer for 1 hour. Check water level occasionally to prevent scalding, adding more as necessary. Stir the oil and sprigs periodically.

3. Using a fine-mesh sieve or several layers of cheesecloth, strain the rosemary leaves from the oil into a pourable container. Discard the herbs.

4. Allow the oil to cool for 10 minutes, and then add the rosemary and lavender essential oils. Stir gently using a wooden chopstick or wooden spoon. Using a funnel, transfer the oil to an 8-ounce bottle and cover the bottle with a lid. Remember to date and label your container.

5. When you're ready to apply the oil, pour about ¼ cup (60 ml) across your scalp. Using your fingertips, massage the oil into your scalp and down the length of your hair, all the way to the ends. If your hair is long, wind it up into a bun and secure it in place with a hair clip after applying. Cover the hair with a shower cap or towel.

6. Leave the oil to infuse for at least 30 minutes, preferably an hour. Alternatively, leave in place overnight, placing a towel over your pillows to avoid staining your pillowcases.

7. Shampoo your hair to wash out the oil thoroughly. Depending on the length of your hair, this may require two washes. Condition and style as usual.

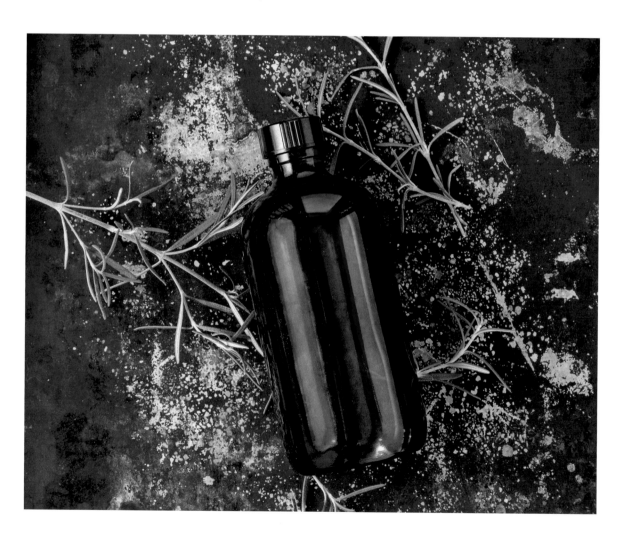

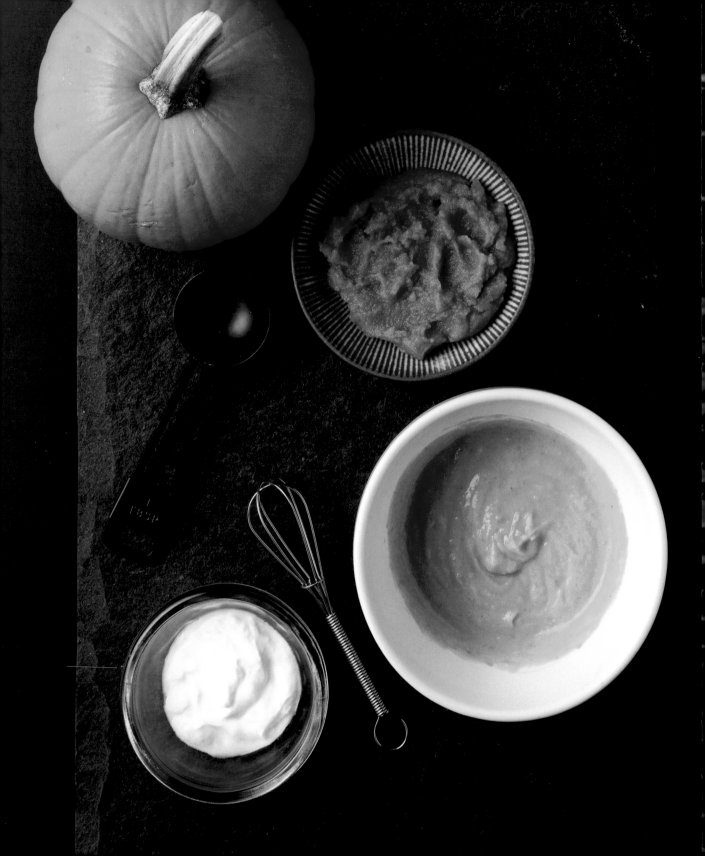

# PUMPKIN MASK

We heat our home almost exclusively with a wood-burning stove. While this makes for a cozy atmosphere and permeates the house with a delicious aroma, it has the unfortunate downside of wreaking havoc on my skin. My husband stacks the wood, brings it in, and feeds it overnight, while I typically feed the stove during the day. All the dry air that hits my face each time I open the stove takes its toll as autumn morphs into winter. When my daily moisturizer alone doesn't seem to offer enough comfort, I turn to this mask. Pumpkin contains numerous nutrients, including alpha hydroxyl acids that facilitate the skin's sloughing process and smooth its surface as it produces new cells. High quantities of vitamins A and C from the pumpkin have skin-smoothing properties as well, and boost collagen production.

Yield: 1 application  •  Frequency of use: Use once weekly.  •  Storage: Do not store. Use immediately.

## » To Prepare:

1. Place the ingredients into a small bowl. Whisk gently until completely combined.

2. Slather liberally on face and neck. If you have long hair, I suggest using a headband to keep it off your face. Leave the mask on for 15 minutes.

3. Rinse the mask off with warm water and then apply your preferred moisturizer.

## » You Will Need:

¼ cup canned or fresh pumpkin puree*

2 tablespoons plain yogurt (whole, low-fat, or reduced fat)

## Tip

For skin that is especially dry or sensitive, add 1 tablespoon raw honey, which is well known for its moisturizing properties, to the pumpkin mixture.

* Make sure you're just using pureed pumpkin here, not pumpkin pie mix.

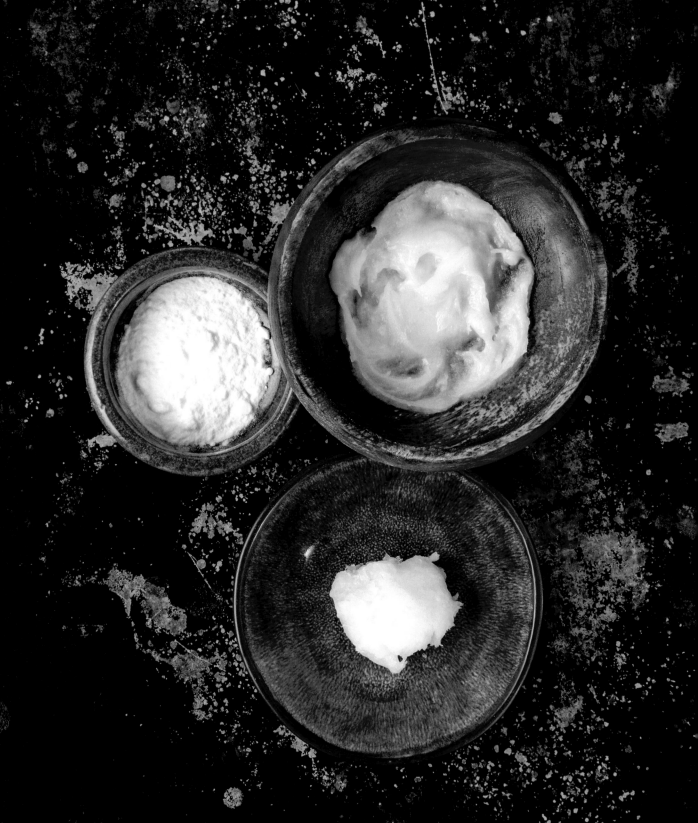

# EASY BAKING SODA EXFOLIANT

As we age, the rate at which our skin naturally produces new cells and sloughs off older ones slows. This partly explains why babies have such soft, tender skin: they haven't aged much yet. Exfoliating helps expedite this process by introducing an abrasive substance to the skin that removes dead cells. Unfortunately, many substances used to exfoliate are too rough, creating more harm than good. That's why I love this simple blend of baking soda and coconut oil. Not only are you likely to have both ingredients on hand already, baking soda is a very mild abrasive that also moisturizes. Plus, it decreases inflammation and balances pH levels, which helps fight acne, redness, and dry skin. Best of all? It only takes seconds to blend together.

**Yield:** 1 application  •  **Frequency of use:** Use once weekly.  •  **Storage:** Do not store. Use immediately.

*Note: If your skin seems to tolerate the exfoliant well, it's fine to add an additional application each week; but take care not to use more than twice weekly, as doing so can irritate the skin. If your skin becomes irritated or feels very taut after use, stick with using it once a week.*

## » To Prepare:

1. Put the ingredients into a small bowl. Using clean hands, mash together to fully combine.

2. Wash your face, removing all makeup. Towel off and apply the exfoliant to your face using a gentle, circular motion, taking care to avoid the eye area.

3. Leave the exfoliant on for 5 minutes and then rinse off with warm water, again avoiding the eye area. Pat the skin dry with a face towel. There shouldn't be any need to apply additional moisturizer, as the coconut oil will have done that job.

## » You Will Need:

2 teaspoons coconut oil

1 teaspoon baking soda

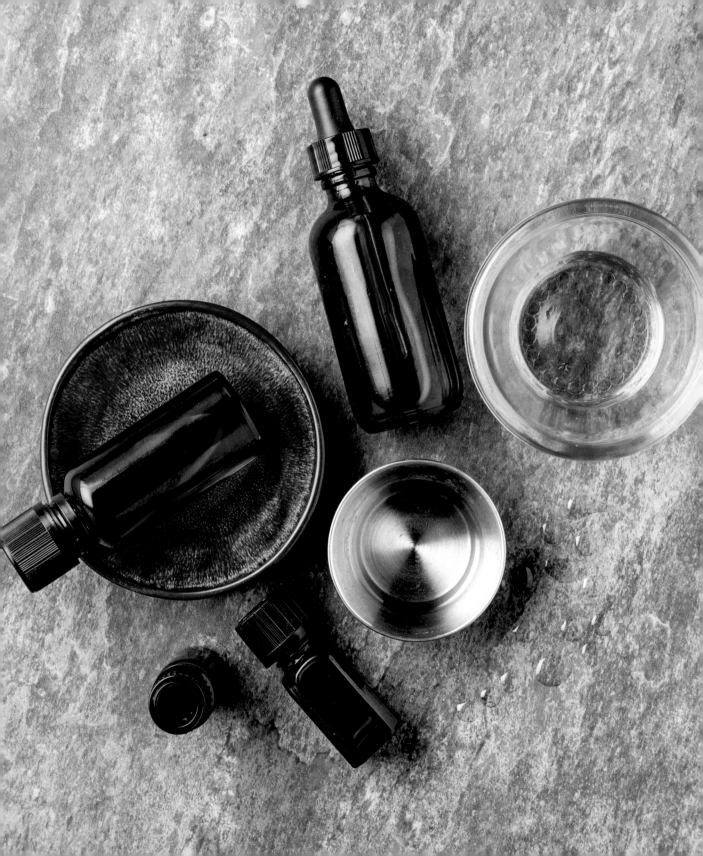

# EVERYDAY FACE OIL

This oil and I are daily acquaintances. My skin tends to be dry, so year-round use of a moisturizer is a necessity. When I began looking into face oils, I was floored by the cost of many off-the-shelf options. After conducting a bit of research on their ingredients, I ultimately created the blend you see here. Both argan and jojoba oil smooth and firm the skin and help with wrinkles and aging, while also offering protection from bacteria and inflammation. Lavender, geranium, and clary sage essential oils are all known for their skin benefits, healing damage, reducing inflammation, and regulating oil production. While my skin tends toward dry, this oil works equally well with all types of skin.

Yield: 2 ounces (60 ml) • Frequency of use: Use daily. • Storage: Store in a cool, dark location, such as a medicine or bathroom cabinet, away from direct sunlight. Use within 6 months.

## » To Prepare:

1. Pour jojoba and argan oils into a 2-ounce (60 ml) glass bottle. Add the remaining ingredients.

2. Place a dropper cap over the bottle, secure, and shake gently to combine fully.

3. To use, dispense about a half dropper-full into the palm of your hand. Apply gently to clean face, taking care to avoid the eyes.

## » You Will Need:

2 tablespoons jojoba oil

2 tablespoons argan oil

2 drops lavender essential oil

2 drops geranium essential oil

1 drop clary sage essential oil (optional)

One 2-ounce (60 ml) glass bottle with dropper cap, preferably blue or amber-colored

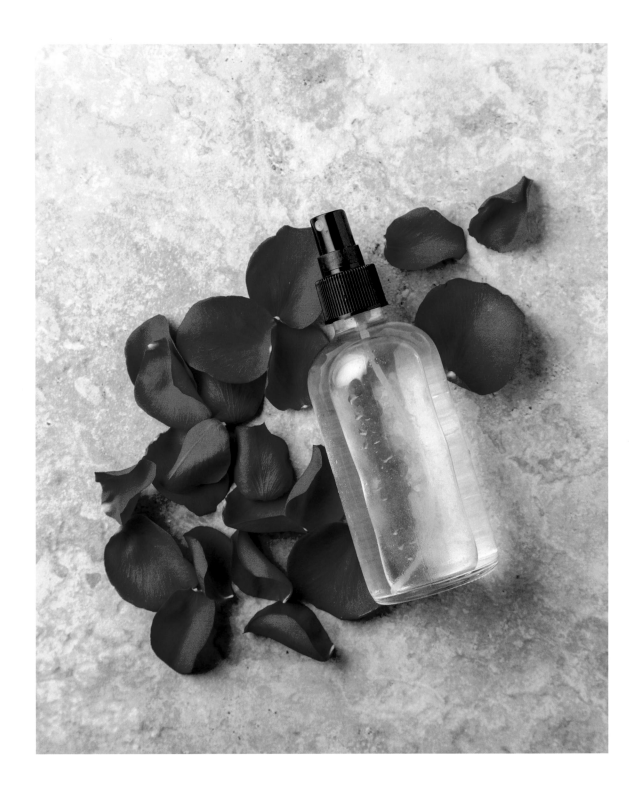

# ROSEWATER TONER

Since I first encountered rosewater while working at a natural foods store in 1997, I have been completely smitten. Its heady fragrance, coupled with its moisturizing and restorative properties, has made it my go-to skin care necessity for decades. Toners help soothe the skin. Because it is used after cleansing the face and just before applying moisturizer, it creates a barrier that locks in moisture. Rosewater helps reduce skin inflammation, an especially useful quality for those who have dry skin or issues such as rosacea, eczema, or acne.

Yield: About 8 ounces (240 ml)  •  Frequency of use: Use daily.  •  Storage: Store in a cool, dark location, such as a medicine or bathroom cabinet. Use within 3 months.

## » To Prepare:

1. Place all the ingredients into a small bowl. Whisk until everything is fully combined. (Alternatively, you can just combine everything in a measuring cup with a pourable spout.)

2. Using a funnel, transfer the toner to an 8-ounce spray bottle. Insert the mister and shake vigorously. Remember to date and label your bottle.

3. To apply, give the bottle a gentle shake, and then spray several pumps across your face, closing your eyes while doing so. Follow with your preferred facial moisturizer.

## » You Will Need:

¼ cup (60 ml) distilled water

¼ cup (60 ml) rosewater

¼ cup (60 ml) witch hazel

1 tablespoon apple cider vinegar

5 drops rosehip seed oil

One 8-ounce (240 ml) spray bottle

# PEEL-OFF CHARCOAL MASK

At least once a month, when the kids are asleep — or, better yet, out somewhere playing with their dad — I treat myself to a hot bath and a charcoal mask. Deeply detoxifying, a charcoal mask is my little treat to myself in the privacy and comfort of my own home. It has exfoliating properties, pulling out anything trapped in your pores and prompting the production of new skin cells. A do-it-yourself, at-home mini-facial — for a fraction of the cost of spa-offered services and none of the questionable ingredients contained in shelf-ready offerings? Yes, please!

Yield: Approximately 4 applications • Frequency of use: Use once every two weeks.
Storage: Store the powered mixture in a cool, dry location. It should be used within 6 months after mixing.

*Note: While deeply cleansing and detoxifying, this mask is also quite drying. Use the mask no more than every two weeks. Don't be alarmed if your skin is red or pink for up to 30 minutes after removing the mask. This is a totally normal side effect of the mask's ingredients and of the process of peeling off the mask.*

## » You Will Need:

4 teaspoons activated charcoal

2 teaspoons bentonite clay

¼ cup (37 g) gelatin powder

2 tablespoons hot (not boiling) water

One 2-ounce (60 ml) glass container

## » To Prepare:

1. Combine the charcoal, bentonite clay, and gelatin powder together in a small bowl. Transfer to the container and cover with a lid.

2. When you're ready to use the mask, remove 4 teaspoons of the powder and place it in a small mixing bowl. Whisk in the hot water until the mixture is smooth.

3. Using clean fingers or a new, unused makeup brush, spread an even layer of the mask across your face. Avoid applying the mask on the delicate skin around your eyes as well as your hairline and your eyebrows, as it will remove any hair it touches when you peel it off. When you finish the application, run the makeup brush, if used, under hot water until the water runs clear, and then set it aside to dry.

4. Allow the mask to completely dry. Depending on how thickly you applied it, this could take anywhere from 10 to 30 minutes.

5. Once the mask has fully dried and feels tight on your face, begin to slowly peel it off. If any areas won't peel off, or if you applied it too close to your hairline or eyebrows, wash it off with warm water instead of attempting to peel it.

6. After you remove the mask, gently splash warm water on your face, and blot dry with a dry washcloth. Apply your preferred facial moisturizer. Discard the mask in the trash, as trying to wash it down the sink could potentially clog the drain.

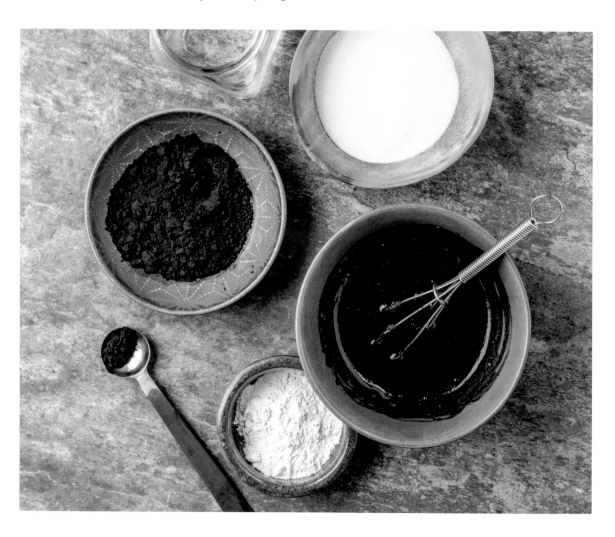

# HONEY BODY SCRUB

Though we often don't think of it as such, our skin is our body's largest organ of elimination. As such, we need to take good care of it, and a body scrub is just the ticket. Sugar gently sloughs off dead, dry skin cells while honey acts as a humectant, pulling in and retaining moisture. Whether you're dealing with dry, leathery skin that's experienced multiple wintertime injustices, or a chlorine-battered body and cracked ankles from summertime escapades, make this honey scrub to use year-round. It'll do its darnedest to soothe whatever ails the skin you're in.

Yield: About 2 cups (540 g), approximately 8–10 applications
Frequency of use: Apply twice weekly. • Storage: Store in a lidded container in a cool, dark location out of direct sunlight. Use within 2 months.

## » You Will Need:

1 cup (200 g) granulated sugar

1 cup (340 g) raw honey

2 tablespoons sweet almond oil or apricot kernel oil

2 tablespoons jojoba oil

5 drops lavender essential oil

One 16-ounce (480 ml) glass container

## » To Prepare:

1. Place all of the ingredients in a medium mixing bowl. Whisk together until fully combined.

2. Transfer contents to the 16-ounce (480 ml) container, cover with a lid, and store in the shower. Remember to date and label your container.

3. Use the scrub during a hot shower. Scoop out several tablespoons at a time. Massage it into your hands, arms, shoulders, back, belly, buttocks, thighs, and calves in a scrubbing motion. Rinse thoroughly, taking care, as the shower floor will be slick. When you're ready, carefully step out of the shower and wipe down any remaining residue on the shower floor. Gently pat your skin dry with a towel.

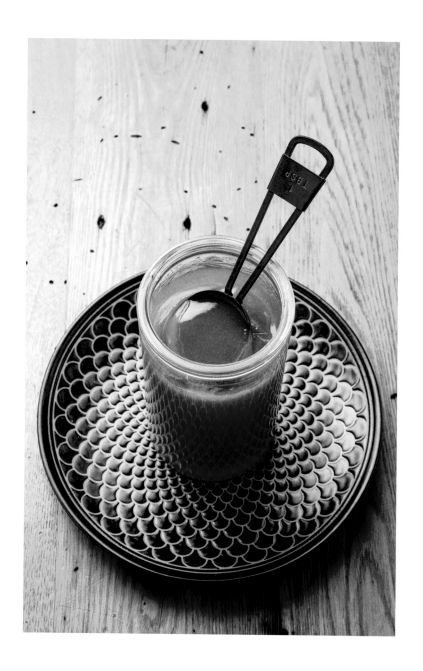

If you suffer from dry lips, this scrub would be a surefire soother! Simply reduce all the ingredient quantities by half, or even by three-quarters, to have a yield of just a wee bit more than 1 cup (300 g), or ½ cup (150 g), depending on how quickly you think you'll go through it.

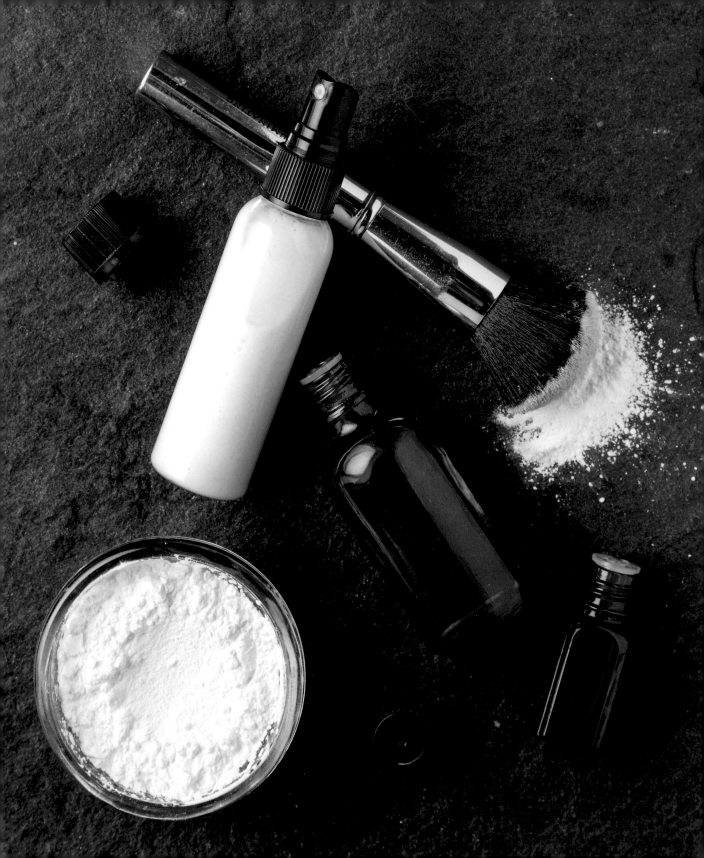

# MILK OF MAGNESIA DEODORANT

When my good friend Adriana, a native of Brazil, told me she'd been using milk of magnesia as a deodorant, I had my doubts — to put it mildly. At the same time, I was also completely intrigued. Turns out, it actually works! I learned that Brazil and other South American countries have long used milk of magnesia as a body odor deterrent. Gentle enough for underarm skin that is sensitive to other natural deodorants (baking soda–based ones make my armpit skin burn horribly), this homemade version was just what I was looking for.

Yield: 2 ounces (60 ml) • Frequency of use: Use daily. • Storage: Store in a cool, dry place, such as a medicine or bathroom cabinet. Use within 1 year.

## » To Prepare:

1. Pour the milk of magnesia into a pourable measuring cup. Add the essential oils and gently whisk together to combine.

2. Using a funnel, transfer the solution to either two 1-ounce glass roller bottles or one 2-ounce glass bottle with a mister. Remember to date and label your container.

3. When ready to use, roll enough of the mixture to cover the armpit area, or mist two or three pumps. After about 1 minute, pour a little bit of arrowroot powder into your hand, and then gently pat it onto both armpits. Alternately, you can apply the arrowroot powder using a designated make-up brush. This will help reduce moisture in addition to odor.

## » You Will Need:

¼ cup (60 ml) additive-free milk of magnesia*

4 drops tea tree essential oil

4 drops lavender essential oil

Arrowroot powder to apply deodorant (optional)

Two 1-ounce (30 ml) glass roller bottles or one 2-ounce (60 ml) glass bottle with mister

* Make sure that the milk of magnesia that you purchase is free of any artificial colors and additives such as xanthan gum, sorbitol, and sodium hypochlorite, which is essentially undiluted bleach.

# PUCKER PACIFIER LIP BALM

I'm an all-day, every-day lip balm wearer. Without it, my lips quickly begin to resemble the Grand Canyon, rife with cracks, ridges, and splits. It's not pretty and not the least bit comfortable. To combat chapped lips, especially when the mercury plummets and the air both indoors and out lacks nearly any form of moisture, I keep myself armed with this moisture-rich lip balm. My blend contains beeswax and coconut oil, which keeps my lips smooth, moisturized, plump, and healthy, no matter what the weather throws my way. It's also a lovely gift to make during the holidays.

Yield: 2 ounces (56 g) • Frequency of use: Apply daily as needed. • Storage: Store out of direct sunlight or intense heat. Best if used within 6 months.

## » You Will Need:

4 tablespoons beeswax, grated or pellets

2 tablespoons coconut oil

5–7 drops essential oil of your choice for scent*

½ teaspoon raw honey or glycerin-based food-grade flavor extracts, such as almond, orange, lemon, etc. (optional)

One 2-ounce (60 ml) glass or metal container

## » To Prepare:

1. Place grated beeswax or beeswax pellets into a heatproof glass dish (one with a spout and handle is ideal). Add coconut oil to the container (the oil will be solid at room temperature).

2. Add 1½ cups (355 ml) water to a small or medium-size pot. Place a silicone trivet or round metal cooling rack in the bottom of the pot. Place the glass dish with beeswax and coconut oil into the middle of the pot, on top of the trivet or cooling rack. Bring the water to a boil. The beeswax and coconut oil will begin to warm and melt. Give the liquid a stir with a metal spoon to fully incorporate the two ingredients.

3. Once melted, remove the glass container from the pot and set it on a kitchen cloth or trivet. Turn the heat off on your stove.

4. Add the essential oil of choice and flavoring agent, if you're using one. Stir with the metal spoon to distribute evenly.

5. Pour the mixture into your container. Cover with a lid. Remember to date and label your container.

6. Allow to fully cool. The mixture will remain solid at room temperature.

*Tip*

For larger batches, simply multiply the ingredient amounts by the number of jars you wish to make. You can also pour the mixture into individual lip balm tubes before it cools.

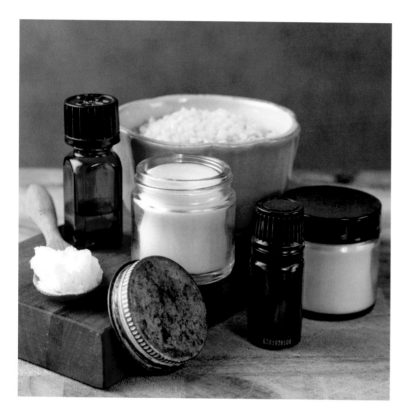

## » Variations

Feel free to experiment with any scent you desire. You can keep it all one fragrance, or you can combine various oils. Whatever you use, use no more than 7 drops total. Here's a list of some of my favorite scent and flavoring combinations, to serve as a springboard for your own creations:

- Peppermint essential oil and orange extract
- Lavender essential oil and lemon extract
- Clove essential oil and orange extract
- Orange essential oil and almond extract
- Spearmint essential oil and lemon extract

# BLISSFUL BATH SALTS

There are few things I love to give to others or receive for myself as much as scented bath salts. They're a simple indulgence that feels so deeply extravagant. Or they do to me, at least! When you're a self-employed, work-from-home mother of two young children, a long, hot soak in the bath is the balm that heals all wounds, literally and figuratively. Making these bath salts couldn't be easier.

Yield: 2½ cups (680 g)  •  Frequency of use: Use 1–2 times weekly.  •  Storage: Store in a lidded container. Best if used within 1 year, as the scents will begin to fade over time.

## » You Will Need:

¾ cup (225 g) Epsom salt

¾ cup (225 g) fine sea salt

1 cup (230 g) baking soda

Essential oils for scent (optional, as follows)

One 24-ounce (710 ml) glass container with lid

### SCENTS:

#### FLORAL BLEND

6–8 drops geranium essential oil

6–8 drops sandalwood essential oil

6–8 drops lavender essential oil

## » To Prepare:

1. Place the Epsom salt, sea salt, baking soda, and optional essential oils into a food processor. Pulse until the mixture is uniform in texture.

2. Transfer the bath salt blend to a covered jar until ready to use. You can place it all in one jar, or use a variety of sizes, especially if you intend to offer any as gifts. Remember to date and label your containers.

3. To use, place around ¼ cup (150 g) into the bath while it's filling. Swirl the water gently to help disperse any bits that might not have dissolved before getting in the tub yourself. Soak for as long as you're comfortable, but aim for at least 15–20 minutes to best receive the benefits of the blend, with 30 minutes being ideal.

## WOODSY BLEND

8 drops fir essential oil

6 drops cedar essential oil

5 drops frankincense essential oil

## CITRUSY BLEND

6–8 drops lime essential oil

6–8 drops lemongrass essential oil

6–8 drops grapefruit essential oil

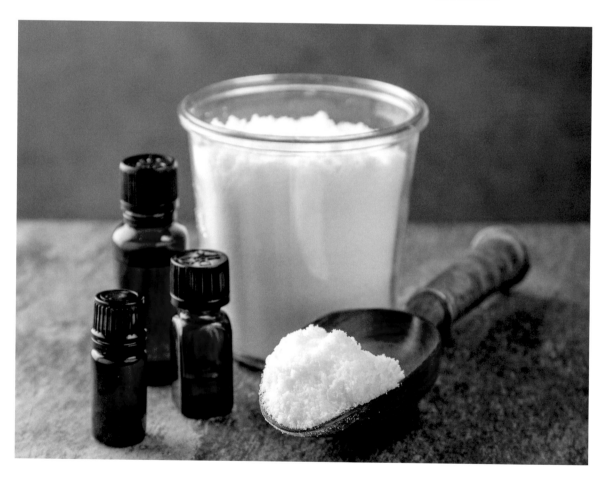

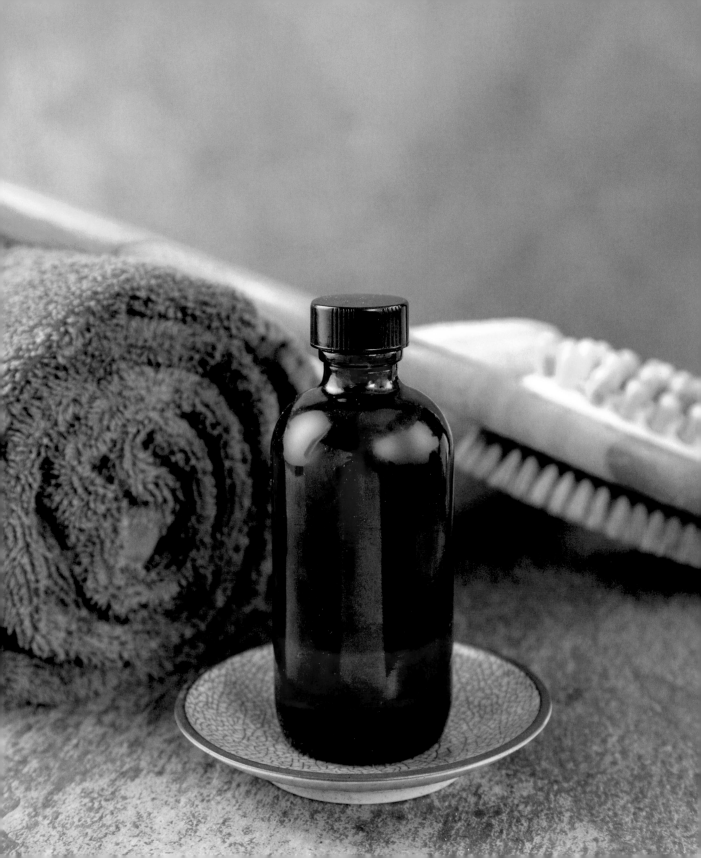

# BATH OIL

While a bath-salt soak calms me, it's a bath-oil soak that nourishes and moisturizes my skin the most. From around late autumn into early spring, I turn to a bit of this oil in my bath to keep my skin happy. Do be mindful that this oil will leave a bit of a slippery coating in the tub, so take great care when entering and exiting, stepping in and out slowly.

Yield: 4 ounces (120 ml) • Frequency of use: Use as needed or desired.
Storage: Store in a lidded container. Best if used within 6 months;
otherwise, the scents will begin to fade and the oils will begin to turn.

## » To Prepare:

1. Place the essential oils into a pourable measuring cup.

2. Add the jojoba and almond oils. Using a funnel, transfer the blend to a dark-colored 4-ounce glass bottle. Remember to date and label your bottle.

3. When ready to use, run your bath. Then add about 1 or 2 tablespoons of the blend and soak for as long as you're comfortable. To avoid slipping, take great caution when stepping out of the bath, and scrub it down afterward to remove all oil residues.

4. Gently pat your skin dry with a towel.

## » You Will Need:

10 drops lavender essential oil

8 drops geranium essential oil

8 drops ylang ylang essential oil

5 drops lime essential oil

2 tablespoons (30 ml) jojoba oil

6 tablespoons (90 ml) sweet almond oil or apricot kernel oil

One 4-ounce (120 ml) tinted glass bottle

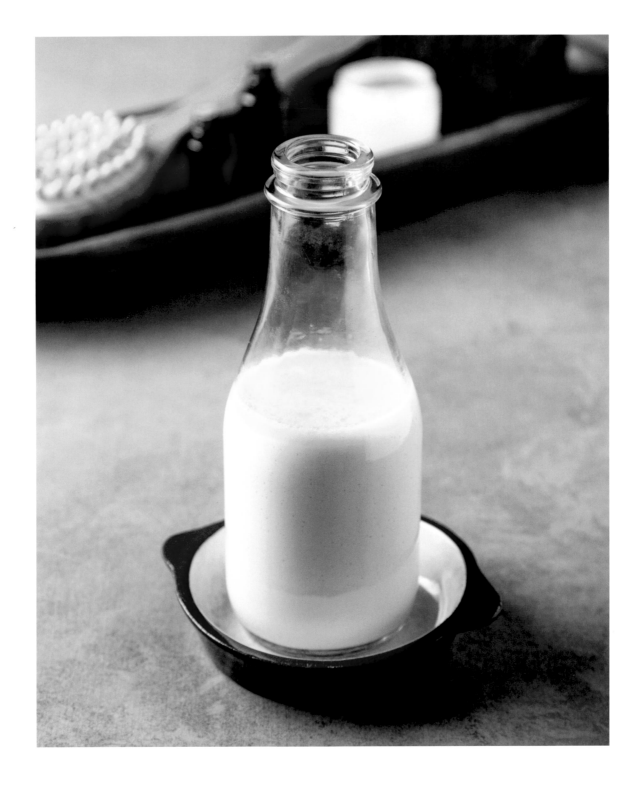

# ROYAL MILK BATH

I think of Cleopatra as the "Notorious KRQ"—kohl-rimmed queen, that is. From her political exploits and romantic relationships to her beauty to her conquests, Egypt's infamous ruler left quite the legacy. She was also well known for her porcelain skin; milk-based baths were purported to be the secret to her enviable visage. But you don't need a crown and scepter to achieve similar results—just open your refrigerator and pantry! The proteins in milk dissolve dead cells on the skin's surface. Honey, also included here, helps seal in moisture. Together, the combination is a full-body skin rejuvenator. You'll emerge from this bath feeling like the royalty you truly are.

Yield: 1 application • Frequency of use: Use as needed, whenever your skin feels especially dry and parched. • Storage: Do not store. Use immediately.

## » To Prepare:

1. In a small pan, gently warm the milk on the stovetop, just until it is the slightest bit warm to the touch. Add the honey and the oils. Whisk until fully incorporated.

2. To use, fill a bath with warm water. Add the milk mixture to the bath. Using your hand, stir the water until the mixture is fully dispersed.

3. Soak as long as the water remains at a comfortable temperature, topping it off with warm water occasionally if desired. To get the most benefit, soak for at least 10–15 minutes.

4. Rinse off with warm water, and gently pat yourself dry with a bath towel.

## » You Will Need:

3 cups (710 ml) milk (preferably whole fat and organic)

2 tablespoons raw honey

2 tablespoons jojoba, sweet almond, or grapeseed oil

5 drops geranium essential oil

# BATH FIZZY

What if you could take a bath that wasn't only relaxing and beneficial to your skin, but also fun? Enter the bath fizzy. It checks off all the boxes for happiness! Baking soda will exfoliate the skin, Epsom salts aid circulation and reduce swelling, and citric acid helps make everything bubble and delight. Individual bath fizzies can cost a good deal of money if purchased off the shelf. That's why I love whipping up a batch of these at home, whether for personal use or for gifting.

Yield: One dozen • Frequency of use: Use as desired. • Storage: Store in a lidded glass jar, or wrap in cellophane, glassine, or parchment bags. Use within 1 year.

## » You Will Need:

1 cup (230 g) baking soda

½ cup (112 g) Epsom salt

½ cup (64 g) cornstarch

½ cup (115 g) citric acid

2 tablespoons canola or safflower oil

1 tablespoon cold water

8 drops essential oil(s) of your choice

5 drops food coloring (optional)

Silicone molds, ¼ cup (60 ml) in volume per mold*

One 32-ounce (946 ml) glass jar

* You'll need to have all your molds accessible during assembly, as the mixture must be pressed into them as soon as you finish mixing it together.

## » To Prepare:

1. Place the baking soda, Epsom salt, cornstarch, and citric acid in a medium bowl. Using a whisk, combine the ingredients thoroughly until no lumps remain.

2. In a small bowl or a pourable measuring cup, whisk together the oils, water, and food coloring, if using.

3. Adding small spoonfuls at a time, whisk the liquid into the dry mixture. Do this very slowly; otherwise the mixture might overfizz and not set properly. Once everything is fully combined, your mixture should be dry, crumbly, and barely sticking together.

4. Scoop about ¼ cup (50 g) into each silicone mold. Press down firmly, and set aside to dry fully. A full day of drying time is ideal.

5. Flip the silicone mold over, and gently release the bath fizzy. Store in your chosen container or wrap it up for gifting. Remember to date and label your containers and packages.

6. To use, fill a bath and drop one bath fizzy into the water. Step in gently, and soak for as long as you're comfortable, refreshing the water as desired. When finished, towel off as usual.

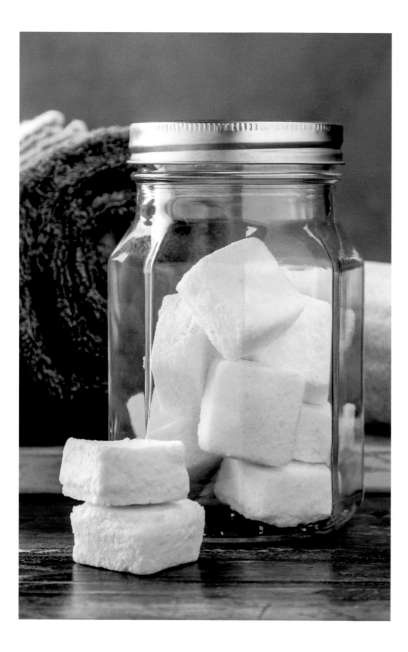

## » Variations

Here's a list of some of my favorite scents for bath fizzies, to serve as a catalyst for creations of your own design:

- Lavender and orange
- Eucalyptus, orange, and ylang ylang
- Fir, juniper, and lemon
- Chamomile and lavender
- Cedar and sandalwood

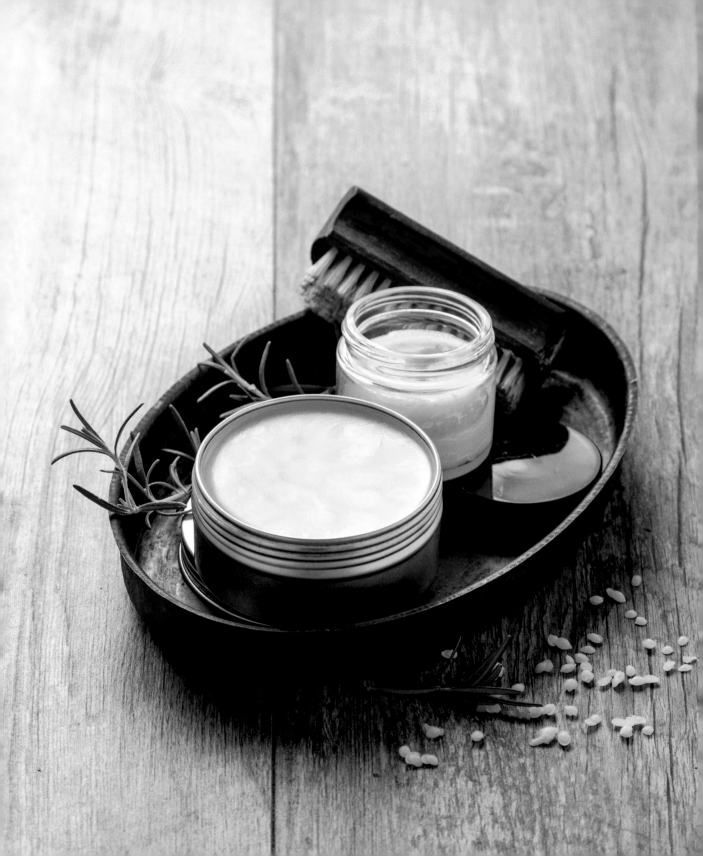

# HAND SALVE

I don't know about you, but my hands are under siege pretty much all year long. From filling the wood stove to hand-washing dishes, the skin on the backs of my hands all the way down to my fingers becomes dry, cracked, and downright painful. Thankfully, a bit of hand salve is all it takes to mend things. Olive oil, beeswax, and coconut lock in moisture, while lavender proves deeply healing to damaged skin. A wee bit of vitamin E oil acts as a natural preservative, keeping the oils from going rancid.

**Yield:** About ¾ cup (180 ml) • **Frequency of use:** Use whenever the weather is dry and cold, or when hands are calloused and could use a bit of TLC. • **Storage:** Store in a cool place out of direct sunlight. Use within 6 months.

## » To Prepare:

1. Place about 2 inches (5 cm) of water in a small pan. Place a silicone trivet or round metal cooling rack in the bottom of the pan. Put a pourable heatproof glass or metal container in the middle of the pan, on top of the trivet/cooling rack.

2. Add the olive oil, beeswax, and coconut oil to the container.

3. Bring the water to a boil, and stir with a wooden utensil until everything has melted. (I use a wooden chopstick to stir.)

4. Once everything has liquefied, remove the pan from the heat. Add the lavender, rosemary, tea tree, and vitamin E oils. Stir to fully disperse. Carefully pour the oil into the container.

5. Once the oil has cooled and solidified, cover with a lid. Remember to date and label your container.

6. To use, scoop out a small amount, about 1 teaspoon, and massage gently into both hands.

## » You Will Need:

10 tablespoons (150 ml) extra-virgin olive oil

¼ cup (57 g) beeswax, grated or pellets

3 tablespoons coconut oil

8 drops lavender essential oil

8 drops rosemary essential oil

8 drops tea tree essential oil

½ teaspoon vitamin E oil

One 8-ounce (240 ml) glass or metal container

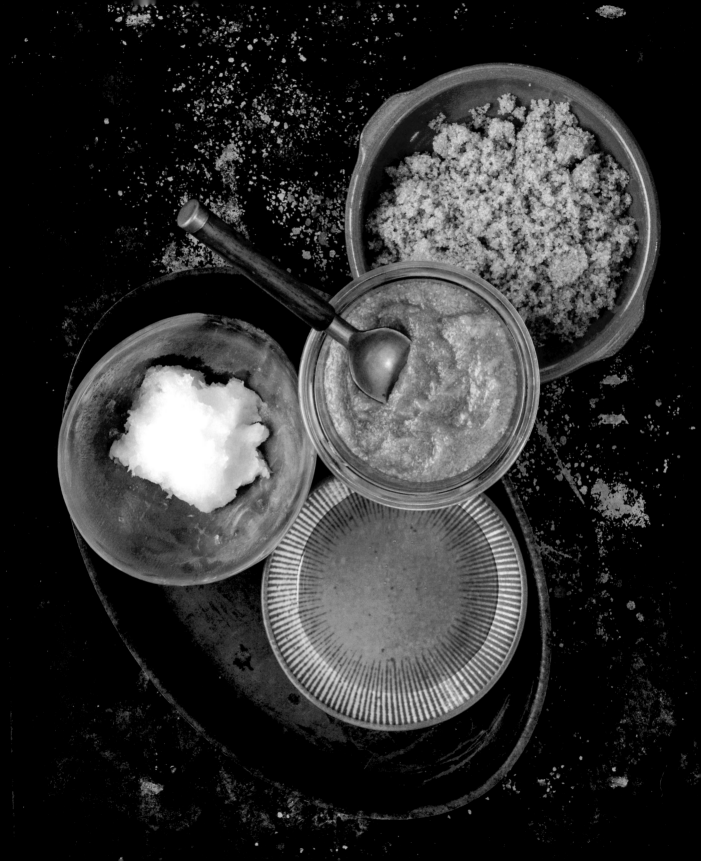

# BROWN SUGAR FOOT SCRUB

Honey isn't just delicious—it's also healing. Antibacterial properties in this sticky substance help expedite wound healing. Using its hygroscopic ability to pull moisture out of wounds, honey curtails bacterial growth in the process. What that means for you, and your feet especially, is that after you enjoy a nourishing bit of honey in your tea, you should slather some onto your tootsies. Our feet endure so much, and tending to them properly is essential. This mixture of brown sugar, coconut oil, honey, and peppermint essential oil will heal, moisturize, and invigorate your body's literal support system.

Yield: About ⅓ cup (80 ml)  •  Frequency of use: Use once every 1 to 2 weeks, as needed.
Storage: Store in a cool place out of direct sunlight. Use within 6 months.

## » To Prepare:

1. Combine all the ingredients in a small mixing bowl. Stir to fully combine. Transfer the mixture to a 4-ounce (120 ml) container, covering it with a lid and remembering to label and date it.

2. To use, massage about ½ tablespoon per foot with firm strokes.

3. Rinse the scrub off with warm water and dry feet completely with a towel. Save any unused portion in your chosen container, covering with a lid.

## » You Will Need:

¼ cup (55 g) brown sugar

2 tablespoons coconut oil

2 tablespoons honey

3 drops peppermint essential oil

One 4-ounce (120 ml) glass or metal container

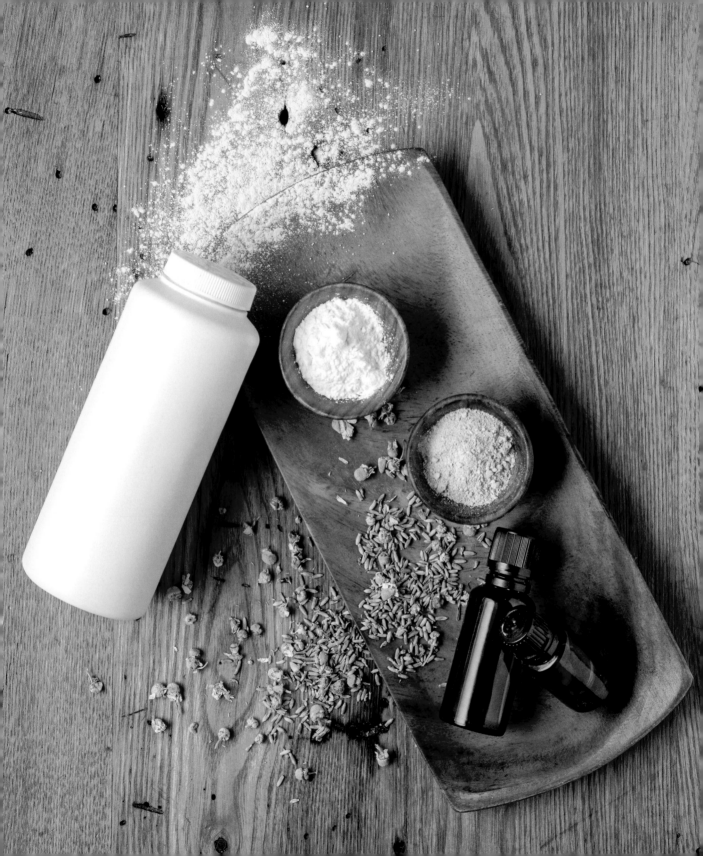

# HIGH & DRY BABY POWDER

Where there are babies and diapers, there is moisture. There's simply no escaping it. Prolonged exposure to moisture, especially from urine, can greatly irritate baby's delicate skin. Baby powder is especially helpful for keeping skin dry, acting as a moisture barrier. I use a bit of it on my children during nearly every diaper change and have had tremendous success in keeping diaper rash at bay.

Yield: 1 cup (128 g)  •  Frequency of use: Apply once per diaper change.

Storage: Store in a lidded container and use within 1 year.

## » To Prepare:

1. Put the kaolin clay, arrowroot powder, and essential oils into a small mixing bowl. Using a whisk, combine thoroughly until the ingredients are fully incorporated.

2. Transfer the mixture to the bottle. Remember to date and label it.

3. To use, gently shake a small amount of powder into the palm of your hand, and then pat it onto baby's skin.

## » You Will Need:

½ cup (64 g) white kaolin clay

½ cup (64 g) arrowroot powder

5 drops chamomile essential oil

5 drops lavender essential oil

One 8-ounce (240 ml) bottle with a shaker top

# BOTTOMS UP DIAPER CREAM

Despite your best efforts, sometimes diaper rash happens. No matter how fastidious you may be at pow-dering and changing a diaper, foods that baby ate might irritate their bellies, resulting in soiled diapers that burn and irritate. This cream will save the day when redness appears. Feel free to divvy it up into smaller portions, using four 2-ounce (60 ml) jars, if you'd like to keep it in a variety of locations, including your diaper bag, changing table, purse, or car. This cream is also helpful for older children experiencing irritation in sensitive skin areas.

Yield: About 8 ounces (240 ml) • Frequency of use: Apply as needed, whenever baby's skin is red or irritated. • Storage: Store in a cool, dark place, and use within 6 months.

## » You Will Need:

½ cup (109 g) shea, cocoa, or mango butter

¼ cup (55 g) coconut oil

2 teaspoons beeswax, grated or pellets

¼ cup (65 g) bentonite clay

8 drops lavender essential oil

6 drops tea tree essential oil

One 8-ounce (240 ml) glass jar or four 2-ounce (60 ml) glass jars

## » To Prepare:

1. Fill a small saucepan almost halfway with water. Place it on the stovetop.

2. Put the shea, cocoa, or mango butter, coconut oil, and beeswax in a heatproof glass jar or pourable measuring cup. Whichever you choose, it should be at least 8 ounces (240 ml) in size.

3. Gently place the jar into the saucepan containing water. The water level should fall a little more than halfway up the side of the jar; if it exceeds that, pour some out.

4. Turn the heat to medium. Over the next 15–20 minutes, stir the contents of the jar around with a wooden spoon or wooden chopstick.

5. Once everything has liquefied fully, remove the pot from heat and carefully remove the jar from the pot using oven mitts. Set the jar on a trivet or cloth on the counter, and leave to cool to room temperature.

6. Once the jar is cool enough to handle, transfer its contents to a medium-size mixing bowl. If the mixture has solidified in the jar as it cools, simply use a spoon or spatula to scoop it out.

7. Add the bentonite clay and the lavender and tea tree essential oils to the mixture. Using a wooden spoon, stir everything together until the clay and essential oils are fully incorporated. Set the mixture aside to firm up. Depending on the temperature inside your home, this may take as little as 1–2 hours or as much as 6–8 hours.

8. Using a spatula, transfer the mixture to a food processor or blender. Process until the blend begins to firm up and stiffen. Transfer the mixture to your chosen container. Remember to date and label it.

9. To use, scoop out about a tablespoon's worth. Apply liberally across diapering area, or wherever redness or rash are present. Repeat at each diaper change until problem areas have disappeared.

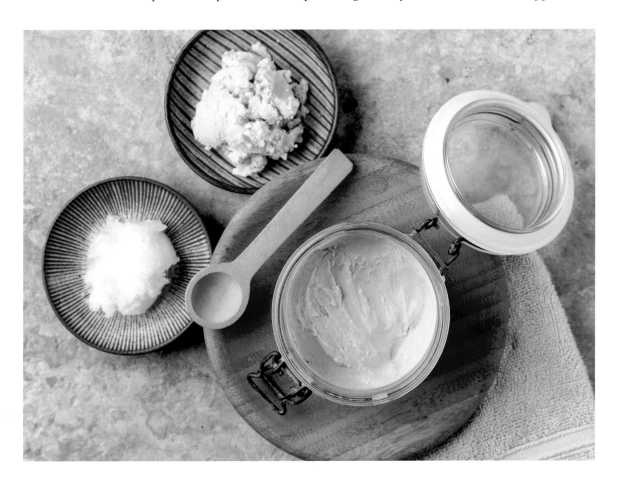

# BABY MASSAGE OIL

My son Alistair was born three months prematurely and went on to spend nearly three months in the hospital. I visited him every day for skin-to-skin "kangaroo" time, a type of direct contact where the baby is dressed in only a diaper and placed on his parent's bare chest to encourage growth and development. One day, I found him in the lap of his physical therapist, Becky. She was gently applying pressure to his hips, shoulders, and all his joints, and he deeply, deeply enjoyed it. Becky encouraged me to continue this practice once Alistair came home. I took her advice and created this oil. He loved receiving massages just as much as I loved giving them. It's such a sweet, tender way of relaxing with your baby.

Yield: 4 ounces (120 ml) • Frequency of use: Use at bed or naptime, or any time baby could use some calming. • Storage: Store in a cool, dry, dark location, such as a medicine cabinet or bathroom cabinet. Use within 1 year.

## » *You Will Need:*

4 ounces (120 ml) sweet almond oil or apricot kernel oil

¼ cup (8 g) dried calendula

¼ cup (8 g) dried chamomile*

5 drops lavender essential oil

3 drops cedarwood essential oil

2 drops ylang ylang essential oil

One 4-ounce (120 ml) dark glass bottle

* *Avoid using the contents of chamomile tea bags, which tend to consist of chamomile flowers that have been cut, sifted, and powdered. You want dried whole flowers here.*

## » *To Prepare:*

1. If you don't already have a double boiler, create a DIY version using the instructions on page 17.

2. Place a metal bowl on top of the water-filled pot. The bowl should be wide enough to fit across the top of the pot, but not deep enough to touch the water in the pot.

3. Put the almond oil and dried herbs into the metal bowl. Reduce the water to a simmer, and leave the oil to infuse for about 45 minutes. Check the water level periodically, topping the pot up with additional water as necessary to keep the level consistent.

4. Line a fine-mesh sieve with muslin, finely woven cheesecloth, or a double layer of paper towels. Place the sieve on top of a medium bowl, and pour the oil into it. Discard the herbs.

5. Place the essential oils into the bottle. Using a funnel, pour the infused oil in. Put a lid on the bottle, and gently tip it from side to side to distribute the essential oils into the infused oil. Remember to date and label your container before storing.

6. To use, pour about ½ tablespoon into the palm of your hand. Rub your hands together to warm the oil, and then gently massage it into baby's skin. This blend is especially useful during bed or naptime, to help induce sleep.

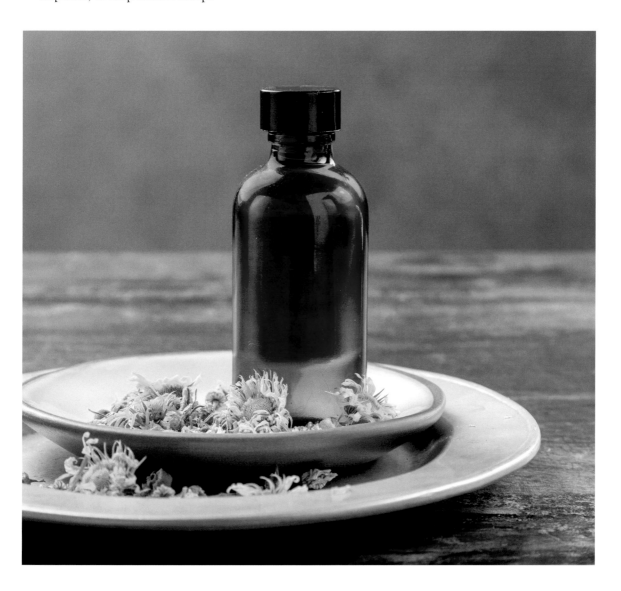

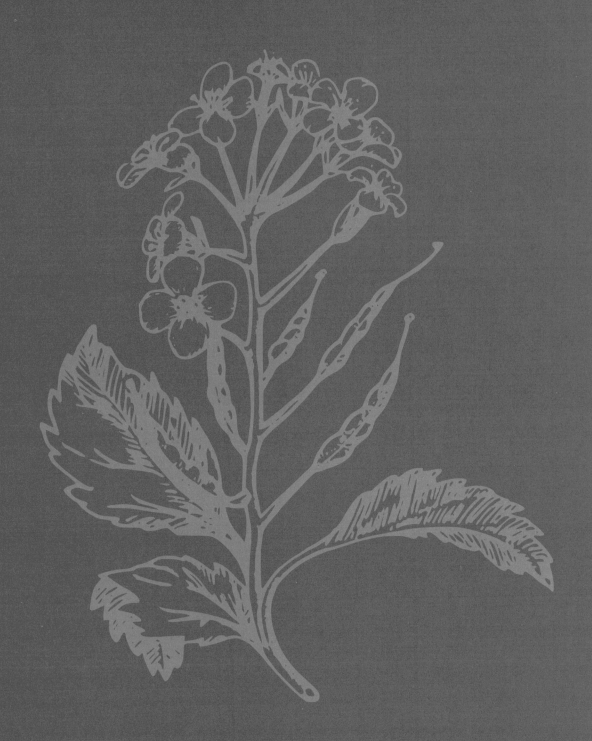

# Natural
# Health

There are few things I find more deeply comforting than knowing that, should illness or injury befall myself or my loved ones, I hold in my power the ability to treat their ailments. To do so in my own home is beyond empowering, and the sense of personal agency it offers is enriching. While I love canning jars of pickles or batches of jam, there's just something about making homemade natural wellness remedies in my kitchen that satisfies my inner nurse-mama-healer like nothing else. You might be surprised to find many of the ingredients for crafting these recipes already in your kitchen or cupboard. Less-common items can be easily sourced online.

# ELDERBERRY & HONEY SYRUP

As soon as the nights start getting cooler and I see the first leaves fall, I cook up a batch of this syrup. It's my family's fall and winter wellness go-to. Rich in antioxidants, elderberries keep the immune system strong by boosting the production of cytokines, proteins that function as messengers that send inflammatory or anti-inflammatory responses depending on what the body signals. Elderberries are also high in antiviral compounds, which help staunch the spread of viruses internally. In addition to helping at the time of year when we need the most immune-boosting we can get, this syrup is also delicious.

Yield: About 2 cups (480 ml) • Frequency of use: For children 12 and older and adults, take 1 tablespoon daily during cold and flu season as a preventative measure. If you're sick, take 1 tablespoon twice daily (once every 6 hours). For children two and older, take 1 teaspoon preventatively, and 1 teaspoon every 6 hours acutely. For children under two, consult your physician before use. • Storage: Refrigerate; use within 3–4 months.

Note: *If you are pregnant or nursing, or have children under the age of 2, you should check with your physician before use. And don't forget that babies under the age of 1 can't consume honey.*

## » You Will Need:

2 cups (480 ml) distilled water

½ cup (73 g) dried elderberries

1 cinnamon stick

1 knob fresh ginger, peeled (about a 1-inch/2.5-cm piece)

1 teaspoon whole cloves

1 cup (240 ml) raw honey

One 16-ounce (480 ml) glass bottle

## » To Prepare:

1. Combine the water, elderberries, and spices in a medium-size saucepan. Bring to a boil.

2. Reduce the heat to low, cover the pot with a lid, and simmer for 20–25 minutes, until the syrup reduces by about half.

3. Remove the saucepan from the heat. Set aside.

4. Fill a bottle with the honey and place a funnel over the bottle. Using a sieve placed over the funnel, strain the syrup

into the honey. Use a spoon to press the berries against the sieve, extracting as much of their juice as possible. Discard or compost the solids.

5. Place a lid on the bottle. Shake vigorously to fully combine the syrup with the honey. Label the bottle with the date and place it in the refrigerator.

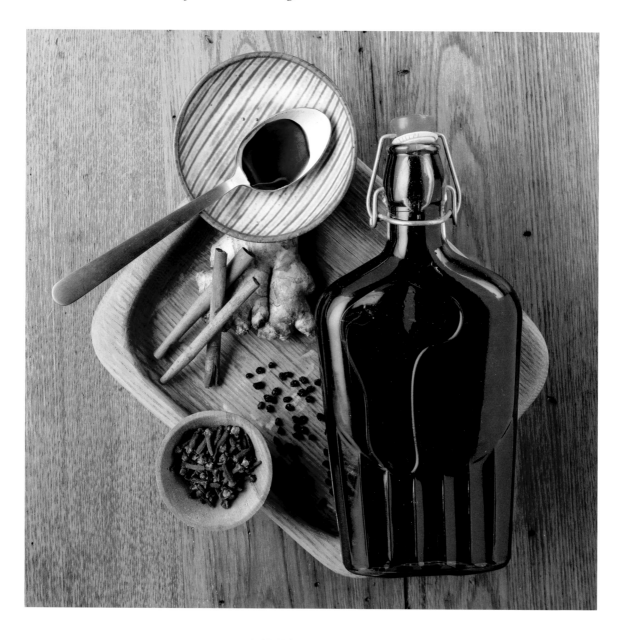

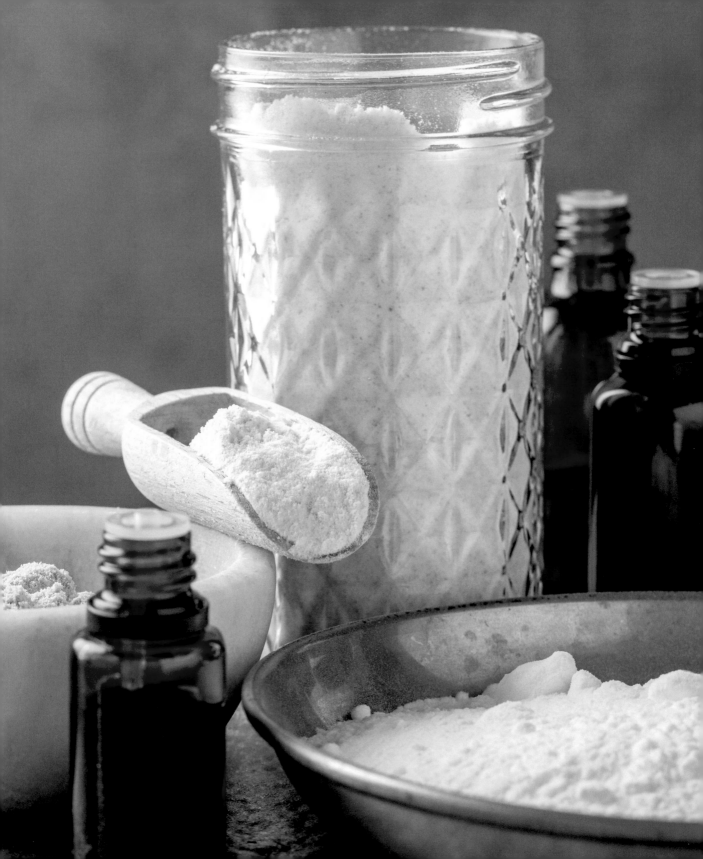

# MUSTARD BATH

Used for centuries by the ancient Greeks and Romans, Native Americans, and practitioners of Ayurvedic medicine, mustard baths are helpful for dealing with colds, stress, sore muscles, fever, and congestion. The mixture used to create the baths contains powdered herbs that have the ability to stimulate sweat glands and increase circulation. This, in turn, helps the body eliminate substances causing it distress or discomfort. I began using mustard baths in my early twenties, when I worked at a variety of natural-food stores and came across a packaged blend formulated by renowned acupuncturist, osteopath, and homeopathist Dr. Shyam Singha. Not only was it effective, but it was invigorating and deeply aromatic to boot. I've modeled my mustard bath on his and hope that it provides just the relief you're looking for.

Yield: Enough for 4 baths • Frequency of use: Use once daily at the first sign of cold or flu, pain, or illness. • Storage: Store in a lidded container in a cool, dry area. Use within 1 year.

## » To Prepare:

1. Using a whisk, combine all ingredients together in the container. Remember to label and date the container.

2. When ready to use, add about 4 tablespoons of the powder to a running bath. Swish the water around with your hands to disperse it. Soak for as long as you are comfortable, topping off with warmer water as needed.

## » You Will Need:

1 cup (230 g) baking soda

¼ cup (26 g) mustard powder

6 drops wintergreen essential oil

6 drops rosemary essential oil

6 drops eucalyptus essential oil

One 10-ounce (292 ml) glass container

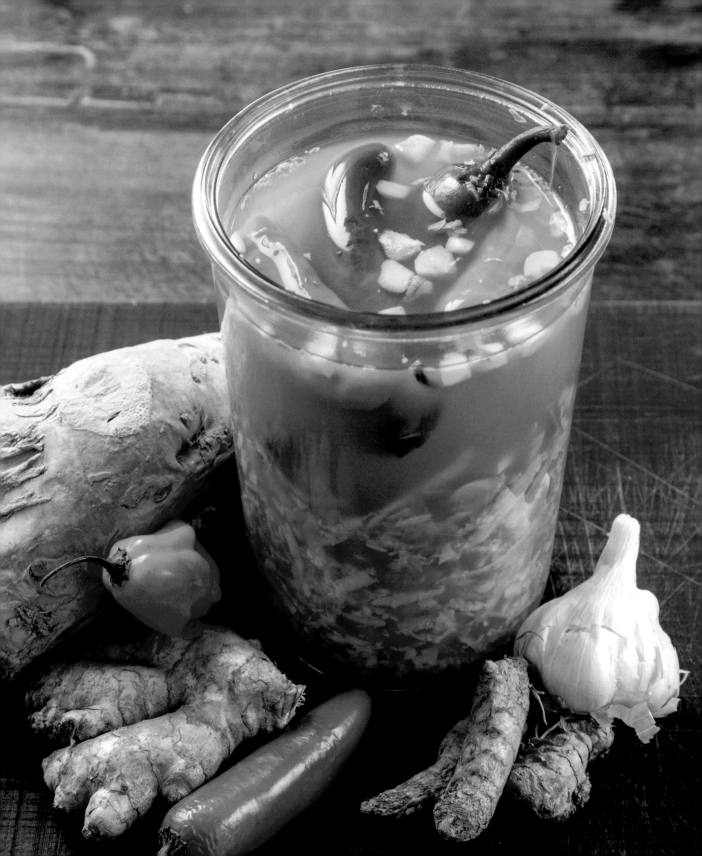

# FIRE CIDER

Fire cider is an infusion of apple cider vinegar; hot, warming herbs such as garlic, horseradish, and ginger; and optional additions including turmeric, ginseng, and hot pepper. Created in the 1980s by renowned herbalist Rosemary Gladstar, this concoction is often used to facilitate the movement of phlegm and congestion. Ever since, herbalists both amateur and professional have been brewing up batches of the cider to get ahead of winter ailments. It takes several weeks to properly infuse, so I encourage you to concoct a jar in the early fall to have it in your arsenal, ready to go, at the first sign of congestion. This is also a great product to have on hand for seasonal allergies. While it won't cure them, it will help alleviate the accompanying congestion.

Yield: 1 quart (950 ml) • Frequency of use: Take 1–2 tablespoons daily preventatively during cold and flu or allergy seasons, or 1–2 tablespoons every 3–4 hours up to four times daily when phlegm and congestion are present. • Storage: Store in a cool, dry location out of direct sunlight. Use within 6 months.

## » To Prepare:

1. Place all the horseradish, ginger, turmeric, garlic cloves, pepper, and ginseng (if using) in a 32-ounce (950 ml) glass container. Pour in the vinegar to cover the ingredients. Cover with a lid, and place in a cool, dark area, such as a pantry or cabinet, to infuse for four weeks. Remember to label the container before storing.

2. Using a fine-mesh sieve, strain the solids. Return the infused vinegar to the glass container and store as before. Discard or compost the solids. Alternatively, you can leave the herbs in, where they'll continue infusing the vinegar, and then strain off the solids upon use.

3. To use, take the fire cider in 1–2 tablespoon doses as needed. Serve sweetened with hot water. I typically put two tablespoons in a mug, top with 1 cup (240 ml) of boiling water, sweeten with several teaspoons of raw honey, and finish with a squeeze of lemon juice.

## » You Will Need:

½ cup freshly grated horseradish

½ cup freshly grated ginger

¼ cup freshly grated turmeric

4 large garlic cloves, minced

2 fresh hot peppers (I typically use cayenne or habanero)

¼ cup chopped ginseng root, fresh or dried (optional)

3 cups (710 ml) apple cider vinegar

Honey and lemon, to serve

One 32-ounce (950 ml) glass container

# HOT HONEY

Every fall and spring, my friend Amanda hosts a handmade swap at her home in North Carolina. Guests arrive with items they have cooked, baked, sewn, brewed, or otherwise made themselves. Offerings range from food to herbal remedies, from framed photographs to body care items, and beyond. I always look forward to attending, and it was at one such gathering that I first encountered hot honey. It's a simple infusion of hot peppers and honey that has been an absolute salvation when colds have decided to set up residence in my nasal passages. The heat from the peppers activates the movement of phlegm, while the honey soothes the throat, a winning combo if there ever was one.

Yield: 2 cups (480 ml) • Frequency of use: Dissolve 1 tablespoon in 1 cup (240 ml) of hot water or tea daily on a preventative basis, or when phlegm and congestion are present, as much as desired. • Storage: Store in a cool, dark area. Use within one year.

*Note: If you are pregnant or nursing, or have children under the age of 2, you should check with your physician before use. And don't forget that babies under the age of 1 can't consume honey.*

## » You Will Need:

3 dried chili peppers, any spicy variety (Cayenne, habanero, jalapeno, Scotch bonnet, and Thai peppers can be used interchangeably here)

2 cups (480 ml) raw honey

One 16-ounce (480 ml) glass jar

## » To Prepare:

1. Place the chili peppers in the bottom of a glass jar. Pour the honey over the peppers.

2. Using a wooden chopstick or the handle of a wooden spoon, stir until the chili peppers are thoroughly coated with honey and fully submerged.

3. Secure a lid to the jar, and leave in a warm, sunny location for seven days. Turn the jar over at least once each day.

4. At the end of the infusing period, warm the honey gently before straining the solids. Place a small pot filled halfway with water over medium heat. Remove the lid from the honey jar and place the jar into the water. The water level in the pot should come no higher than halfway up the jar. Remove excess water as necessary.

5. Gently warm the honey. Stir the honey with a chopstick or wooden spoon handle as it warms, to ensure that the heat is evenly distributed. Take care to not heat it over 110°F (43°C). Use a candy thermometer if you want to be absolutely certain of the temperature. Otherwise, place the jar against your wrist; you should be able to hold it there comfortably for several seconds. Think "baby bottle" warm.

6. Pour the warmed honey over a fine-mesh strainer set atop a clean glass jar. Remember to label the container. Discard or compost the chili peppers, cover the jar with a lid, and store in a cool, dark area.

*Tip*

Hot honey is delicious (and just as therapeutic!) served with food. Drizzle it over chicken (roasted, grilled, fried — it all works equally well), roasted broccoli or brussels sprouts, grilled shrimp or fish, or anywhere else a bit of spicy sweetness would be welcome.

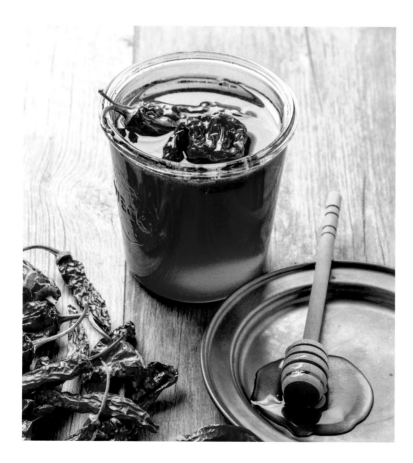

# FULL STEAM AHEAD INHALATION

I will never forget the week I lost my sense of smell and taste. What began as a normal head cold quickly turned into a complete obstruction of my nasal passages. After five days without smelling or tasting anything, a terrifying condition given that my work depends almost entirely on those senses, I turned to my friend Maria. Professionally trained as both a nurse and an herbalist, Maria quickly assembled a package of wellness items and rendezvoused in town with my husband Glenn to transfer it to me. Along with nourishing soup and herbal tinctures, she also instructed me to perform a steam inhalation — cloaking the head with a towel and breathing in hot water infused with herbs or essential oils. Within a day, I could taste, smell, and breathe deeply again.

Yield: 1 inhalation  •  Frequency of use: Use up to three times daily.
Storage: Do not store. Use immediately.

## » You Will Need:

6 cups water

2 drops eucalyptus essential oil

2 drops peppermint
essential oil

2 drops wintergreen
essential oil

1 medium-size bath towel

## » To Prepare:

1. Place the water in a medium pot. Warm over medium-low heat, just until steam begins rising from the surface. Remove the pot from the heat source before any bubbles form.

2. Gather up the bath towel and a bowl large enough to hold all the water. Set the bowl on a table, placing either a kitchen towel or pot holder underneath for stability.

3. Pour the hot water into the bowl. Add the eucalyptus, peppermint, and wintergreen essential oils.

4. Position your head over the bowl and drape the towel over the back of your head, across your shoulders, and over the bowl, creating a sort of tent.

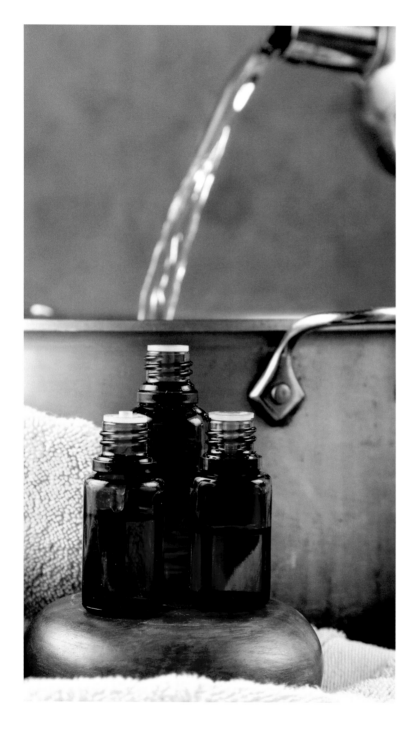

5. Stay in this position for 10 minutes, keeping your eyes closed. (It might be helpful to set a timer right before you drape the towel over your head.) Alternate between breathing through your nose and mouth. You should begin to feel your nasal passages open right away.

6. If your sinuses close up again, feel free to repeat this entire process up to two additional times daily, making a fresh batch of water and essential oil solution each time.

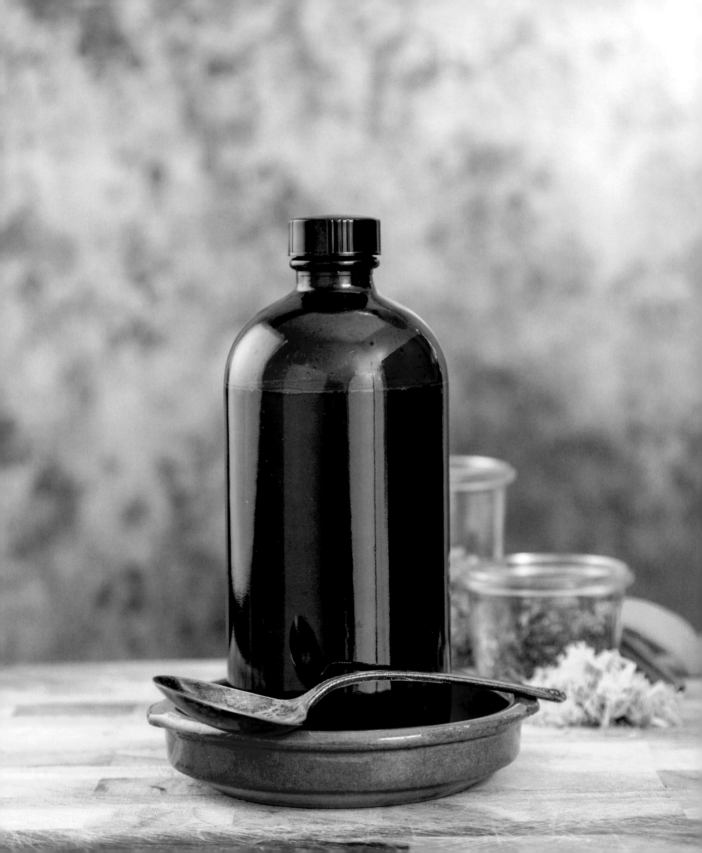

# CATCH YOUR BREATH COUGH SYRUP

Few things are harder to bear than a lingering cough, especially when it's a persistent one that keeps you or your loved ones up at night. The herbs in this syrup help provide a mucilaginous (meaning slippery and gel-like) coating to the throat, and it has antibacterial and anti-inflammatory properties. The syrup keeps for a few months in the refrigerator, so whip up a fresh bottle at the start of each cold and flu season. With a bit of planning and foresight, you'll have a tasty, effective, and economical cough remedy on hand for when the time comes, crafted in your own kitchen without any need to cough up a lung to make it.

Yield: About 2 cups (480 ml) • Frequency of use: For children age 12 and over and adults, take 2 teaspoons every 2 hours as needed, up to four times a day. For children ages 4–12, take 1 teaspoon every 2 hours, up to four times a day. For children ages 4 and under, consult your physician before use. • Storage: Store in the refrigerator. Use within 3 months.

## » To Prepare:

1. Place the water, fennel seed, slippery elm bark, wild cherry bark, cinnamon stick, and orange peel in a medium pan. Bring to a boil over medium-high heat. Reduce the temperature to low, cover with a lid, and simmer gently for 30 minutes, or until the liquid reduces by about half.

2. Remove the pot from the heat. Strain the solids using a fine-mesh sieve, and discard or compost.

3. Place the liquid in a mixing bowl and add the honey. Whisk to fully combine.

4. Transfer the syrup to an amber-colored bottle. Remember to label the container before storing. Cap tightly, and refrigerate.

## » You Will Need:

2 cups (480 ml) cold water

4 tablespoons fennel seed

2 tablespoons slippery elm bark

2 tablespoons wild cherry bark

1 cinnamon stick

Peel from one orange (preferably organic)

1 cup (240 ml) raw honey

# DECONGESTANT BALM

This balm is one of my favorite remedies for stubborn colds, coughs, and congestion. It's a cinch to make, and it smells wonderful. Most importantly, it's effective in opening up the nasal passages. This particular combination of essential oils possesses anti-inflammatory properties, helping to open up airways and bronchial passages.

**Yield:** 2 ounces (57 g) • **Frequency of use:** When sinus congestion is present, apply up to four times daily. • **Storage:** Store in a cool, dark place and use within 1 year.

*Note: This blend doesn't include eucalyptus, making it safe for children 2 years of age or older to use. However, it shouldn't be used in children under the age of 2, as it can encourage mucus production at a rate greater than their narrow air passages are capable of safely expelling.*

## » You Will Need:

¼ cup (55 g) coconut oil

1 tablespoon beeswax, either grated or as pellets

5 drops spearmint essential oil

3 drops spruce essential oil

3 drops fir essential oil

3 drops lavender essential oil

One 2-ounce (60 ml) tin or glass container

## » To Prepare:

1. Place a heatproof glass container such as a mason jar or glass measuring cup inside a medium-size pot. Fill the pot with water until it reaches halfway up the side of the glass container.

2. Put the coconut oil and beeswax into the glass container. Turn the heat to medium. Use a wooden chopstick or the handle of a wooden spoon to stir the mixture, until both the coconut oil and beeswax have fully melted.

3. Remove the pot from the heat. Carefully remove the glass container from the pot and set it on a kitchen towel or pot holder.

4. Add the spearmint, spruce, fir, and lavender essential oils to the liquid mixture. Stir until the oils are fully combined with the beeswax mixture.

5. Pour the mixture into a 2-ounce (60 ml) tin or glass container. Remember to label the container. Set aside to firm up.

6. To use, spread a liberal amount on the chest and then cover with a loose-fitting top. Alternately, spread onto the bottoms of the feet and cover with clean socks before bedtime. The soles of your feet and the palms of your hands lack sebaceous glands, so the oils can permeate your epidermis and start working inside your body much more rapidly than if you applied it elsewhere. Keep the balm away from the face.

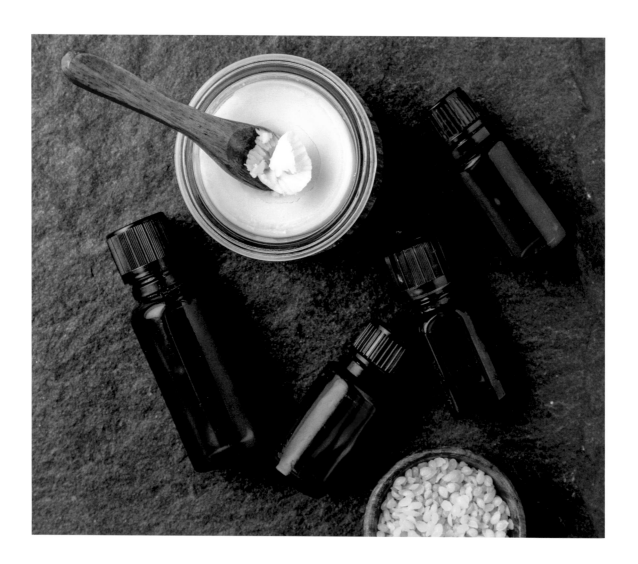

# SOOTHING SPICED COUGH DROPS

I am never without cough drops or breath mints. I try to keep both in my bathroom medicine cabinet and purse at all times. While store-bought versions are certainly convenient, I suggest making a homemade version if you have the time. The fresh ingredients give them a long shelf life and taste better than the average cough drop. The combination of herbs and essential oils helps reduce inflammation in the bronchial passages and throat, while soothing irritated mucous membranes.

Yield: Several dozen • Frequency of use: Use as needed, up to six times daily.

Storage: Store in lidded container in a cool, dry location. Best if used within 3 months.

## » You Will Need:

Powdered sugar, cornstarch, or arrowroot

1 cup (240 ml) distilled water

2 tablespoons dried peppermint

2 tablespoons rubbed sage

One 2-inch (5.1 cm) cinnamon stick

1 tablespoon freshly grated ginger

1 cup (240 ml) raw honey

2 drops clove essential oil

2 drops eucalyptus essential oil

Lidded container for storage, or wax paper or parchment paper for wrapping

## » To Prepare:

1. Place a 9 × 13–inch (23 × 33 cm) baking pan (or similarly sized pan) on the kitchen counter. Sift the powdered sugar, cornstarch, or arrowroot powder to remove any lumps. Pour it across the bottom of the pan until it forms a ½-inch-tall (1.3 cm) layer.

2. Using the bottom of a small food-coloring container or a small spoon, make indentations across the surface of the powder. These will be the "wells" you'll fill up with syrup to create individual cough drops. Set the pan aside and prepare the syrup.

3. Bring the water to a boil in a small pot. Once boiling, remove the pan from the heat, and add the peppermint, sage, cinnamon stick, and ginger. Cover with a lid and leave to infuse for 10 minutes.

4. Strain off the herbs using a fine-mesh sieve or layer of cheesecloth, reserving the liquid. Discard or compost the herbs.

5. Give the pot a quick rinse under cold water to remove any herbal residue, and return it to the stovetop. Add the infused liquid and the honey. Warm over medium heat, stirring occasionally, until the mixture begins boiling. Stop stirring when it starts to boil.

6. Using a candy thermometer, continue boiling until the temperature reaches the hard crack stage, right around 300°F (149°C). Don't get distracted, as the temperature can spike easily, especially once it gets above 290°F (143°C). Remove the pan from the heat.

7. Set the pan aside to cool for 10 minutes, and then stir in the clove and eucalyptus essential oils, using either a wooden spoon or a chopstick. The syrup should now begin to thicken but not harden.

8. Using a spoon, place small spoonfuls of the syrup into the indentations in the powder. Leave to cool for about 1 hour.

9. Once cooled and hardened, toss the drops around in the powder. You want them well-coated on all sides, so really get them moving in there. Remove each drop and either store together loose in a lidded container, or wrap each drop individually in small squares of wax or parchment paper. Remember to label the container before storing.

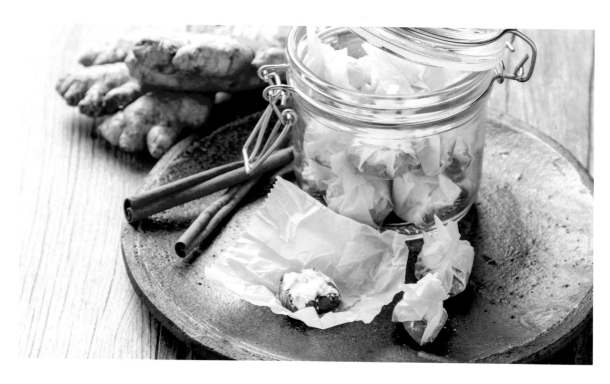

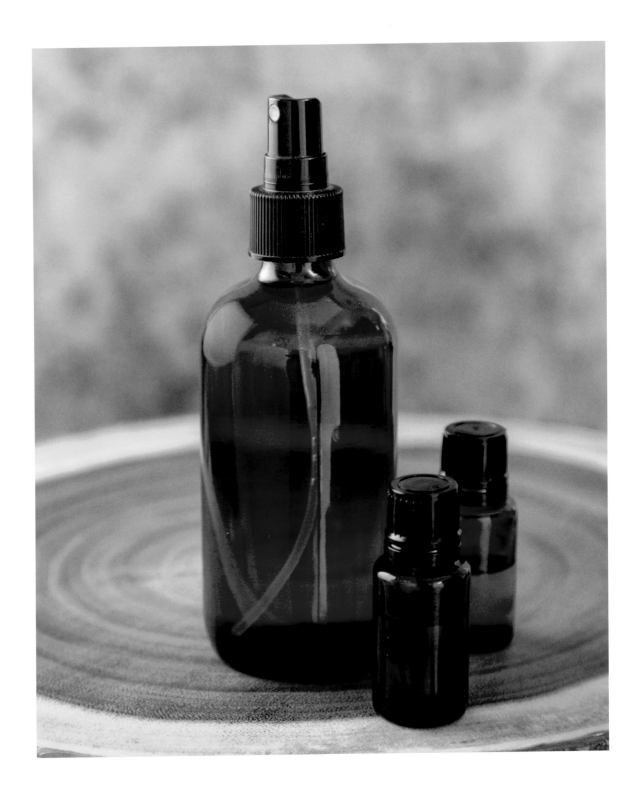

# BUGS AWAY INSECT REPELLENT

Aside from a torrential downpour or dangerous thunderstorm, few things can put a worse damper on outdoor fun than insect bites. You're in the great outdoors, doing your thing, loving life, when a mosquito comes along and rains on your parade, upending your happiness. Get ahead of bites and stings with this insect repellent. I try to keep a bottle at home as well as in the car or my purse all summer long for impromptu outings. Customize the scent to your liking, using a standalone fragrance or a blend created from the bug-repelling essential oils listed below.

Yield: 1 cup (240 ml) • Frequency of use: Use as needed, spraying over the entire body. Repeat application every 2 hours when outdoors. • Storage: Store in a lidded container. Use within 1 year.

## » To Prepare:

1. Place all ingredients into a spray mister bottle. Shake well.

2. To use, spray liberally over any exposed skin before venturing outdoors. Reapply if you get wet or are sweating heavily.

## » Variations

If you need ideas for scent combinations, here are some of my favorite essential oils:

- Lavender and tea tree
- Citronella and lemon
- Rosemary and tea tree
- Citronella, rose geranium, and lavender
- Tea tree, lemon, and rose geranium

## » You Will Need:

1 cup (240 ml) grain alcohol, vodka, or witch hazel

25 drops essential oil(s); select from lavender, citronella, rosemary, rose geranium, lemon, or tea tree oil*

* If you have a preference for a particular aroma, you can use just one single essential oil. You can also try a combination of two or three, or a mixture of all the oils listed.

# BOO BOO GOO

Have this blend of powerhouse ingredients on hand at all times! Coconut oil and lavender are both antibacterial and antimicrobial, while supple olive oil is moisturizing. Historically associated with the healing of wounds, herbs comfrey and calendula fight infection and accelerate immune response. Tea tree is a renowned antiseptic. I carry a mini batch of Boo Boo Goo in my purse for emergency situations, a frequent occurrence when you're the mother of wild, adventurous, free-spirited little ones.

Yield: About 4 ounces (120 g) • Frequency of use: Apply a small amount to minor scrapes and scratches and cover with a bandage. Repeat whenever you change the bandage, up to three times daily. • Storage: Store in a cool, dry location out of direct sunlight. Use within 6 months.

*Note: Avoid using on deep wounds; instead, consult a physician.*

## » You Will Need:

¼ cup (55 g) coconut oil

¼ cup (55 g) extra-virgin olive oil

¼ cup (8 g) dried comfrey

¼ cup (8 g) dried calendula

2 tablespoons beeswax, grated or as pellets

8 drops lavender essential oil

8 drops tea tree essential oil

One 4-ounce (120 ml) glass or metal jar*

## » To Prepare:

1. Place the coconut and olive oils, comfrey, and calendula in a small pot. Warm over medium heat for 15 minutes, stirring occasionally with a wooden spoon or chopstick.

2. Strain the herbs using a fine-mesh sieve or a cheesecloth-lined colander. Discard or compost the herbs.

3. Return the melted oil to the pot. Place over medium heat and add the beeswax. Stir until the beeswax is completely melted and fully incorporated into the oils. Remove the pot from the heat.

4. Add the lavender and tea tree essential oils to the liquid. Stir with your wooden spoon or chopstick until fully blended.

* *You can also use two 2-ounce (60 ml) jars or four 1-ounce (30 ml) jars.*

5. Pour the mixture into whatever container(s) you'd like to use, based on your particular needs. Remember to label your containers before storing. Set aside to cool and firm up.

6. To use, apply about ½ teaspoon to scrapes, scratches, or minor cuts. Cover loosely with a bandage.

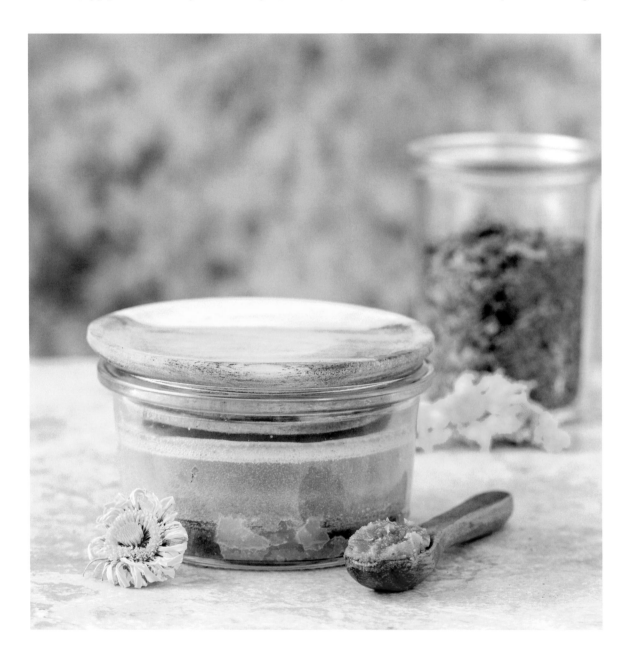

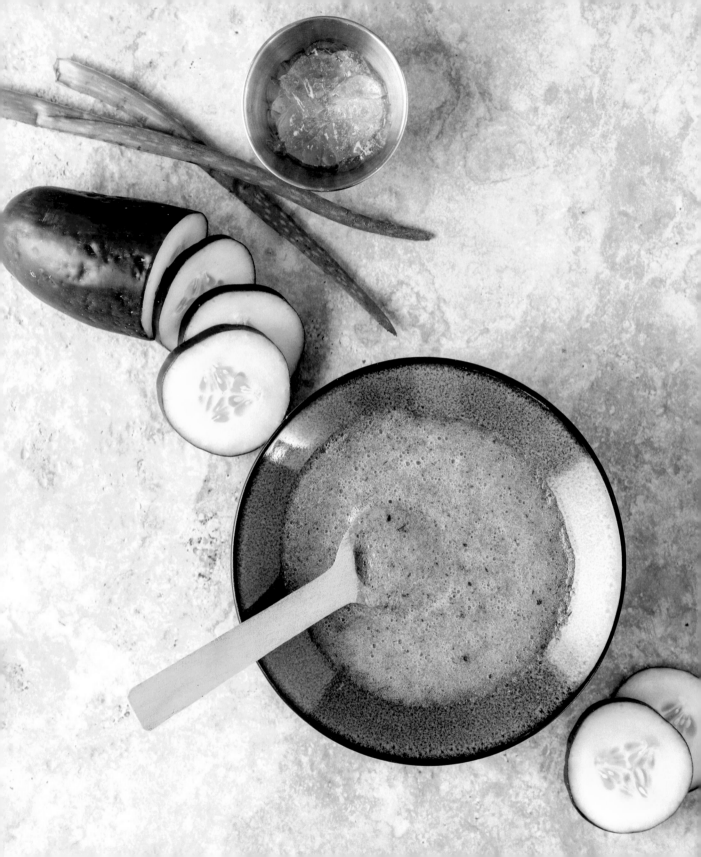

# SUNBURN SOOTHER

To paraphrase Mark Twain, "a cat only sits on a hot stove once." To that, I'd add "a person having the misfortune of experiencing sun poisoning will never experience it again." During a spring-break trip to Miami as a college freshman, I took the overcast skies to mean sunscreen wasn't necessary. Was I ever wrong! Within hours, my boyfriend at the time and I both received full-body sunburns. We were vomiting and barely able to stand upright. These days, I'm the lady under the umbrella, slathered liberally with sunscreen, and wearing a sunhat (or, more likely, avoiding the sun altogether between the hours of 10 and 3). Should you or your loved ones find yourself a bit too pink or red, this all-natural sunburn soother is highly effective.

Yield: 1 application • Frequency of use: Repeat application up to twice daily.
Storage: Do not store. Use immediately.

## » To Prepare:

1. Place all the ingredients in a blender or food processor, and blend until completely smooth.

2. To apply, use clean fingertips to spread the mixture over the sunburned area.

3. Leave the mixture on for 20 to 30 minutes. You may want to wrap up the sunburnt area in an old sheet or large towel so you can sit or lie down and relax.

4. To remove, rinse well with cool water and pat your skin with a dry towel. Apply your preferred moisturizer, and keep the area out of sunlight for at least 1 or 2 days.

## » You Will Need:

¼ cup (57 g) aloe vera gel, store-bought or from a plant

½ cup (67 g) chopped cucumber, with peel and seeds

5 drops lavender essential oil

## Tip

If the area of sunburn is large, you might want to double or triple the ingredient quantities.

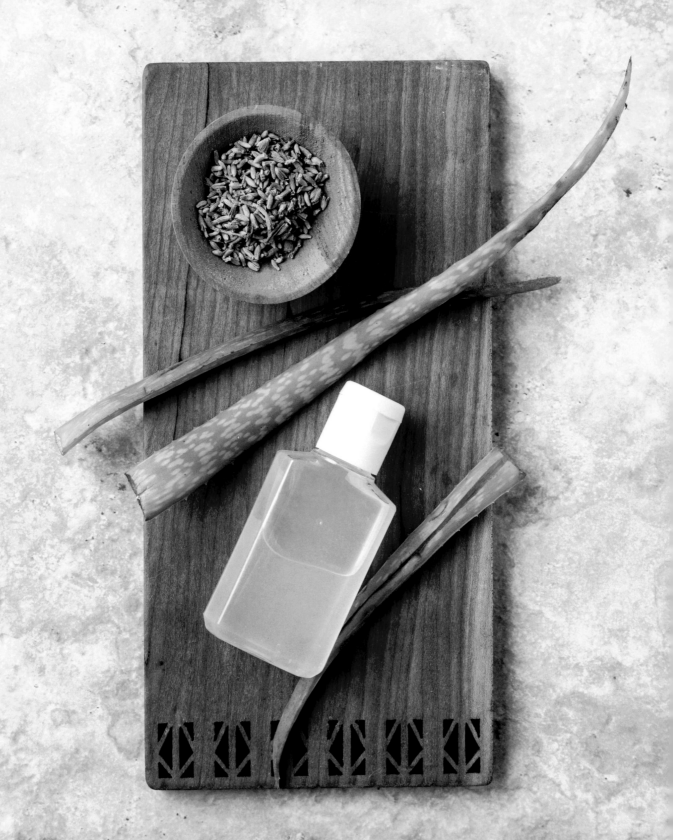

# GERM-BUSTING HAND SANITIZER

When my son Alistair came home after a long stay at the neonatal ICU, he was accompanied by words of extreme caution: the nurses and neonatologists advised me to wash and sanitize my hands when visiting public places, if we couldn't avoid them entirely. You'd better believe I kept hand sanitizer with me at all times. We'd spray on some every time we went into and out of the grocery store, big-box retailers, restaurants, the mall—any kind of indoor public spot. This homemade offering is gentle, nontoxic, and fragrant, and can be made in minutes. The lavender and tea tree oils it contains are both known for their antibacterial and antimicrobial properties.

Yield: 2 ounces (60 ml)  •  Frequency of use: Apply as desired whenever you're out in public places or around those who are sick.  •  Shelf life: Use within 1 year.

## » To Prepare:

1. Place all ingredients in a small bowl. Whisk together until fully combined.

2. Using a funnel, transfer the mixture to a 2-ounce (60 ml) spray or squeeze bottle. Remember to label the container before storing it.

3. Use about a dime-size amount as needed, applying onto one palm and then rubbing both hands together vigorously.

## » You Will Need:

3 tablespoons aloe vera gel, store-bought or from a plant

2 tablespoons vodka (preferably organic)

10 drops lavender essential oil

10 drops tea tree essential oil

One 2-ounce (60 ml) spray or squeeze bottle

# SLEEP SALVE

While many of us drift off to sleep as soon as our heads hit the pillow (thankfully raising my hand), sleep is far more elusive for others. Whether you have a mind that races once you turn the lights out, insomnia, or wiggly, rambunctious children you're trying to get down for the night, I highly recommend dabbing a bit of this salve on yourself at bedtime. The essential oils used here all have antianxiety properties, while lavender has sedative properties. It's based on a blend my dear friend Wendy made years ago, back in my days working as a medical assistant and nutrition consultant for an integrative medicine doctor in Asheville.

Yield: 2 ounces. • Frequency of use: Apply nightly, or at naptime. • Storage: Store in a cool, dry location out of direct sunlight. The salve is most potent within 6 to 8 months of making it.

## » You Will Need:

3 tablespoons extra-virgin olive oil

1 tablespoon sesame oil (not toasted)

1 tablespoon beeswax, grated or pellets

15 drops lavender essential oil

10 drops tangerine essential oil

10 drops sandalwood essential oil*

10 drops coriander essential oil (optional)

One 2-ounce (60 ml) glass, metal, or ceramic container

* You can substitute an equal amount of ylang-ylang, neroli, or chamomile essential oil for the sandalwood.

## » To Prepare:

1. Place a heatproof glass container, such as a Pyrex measuring cup or a mason jar, inside a small pot. (I prefer using a spouted container for this, as it makes pouring easier; but any type made of heatproof glass will work.)

2. Fill the pot with 1–2 inches (2.5–5.1 cm) of water, until it is halfway up the side of your glass jar.

3. Put the olive oil, sesame oil, and beeswax in the glass jar. Bring the water to a gentle boil.

4. Using a wooden stirrer, such as a chopstick, stir the oils around gently until they have fully melted.

5. Remove the pot from the heat. Add the essential oils to the melted oil blend. Gently stir with your wooden utensil until the essential oils are completely incorporated.

6. Pour the oil mixture into the container. Allow it to cool, then cover the container with a lid and label them.

7. At bedtime, rub the salve into your temples and onto your forehead, and dab a bit under your nose. You can also put some on the backs of your hands and onto your wrists.

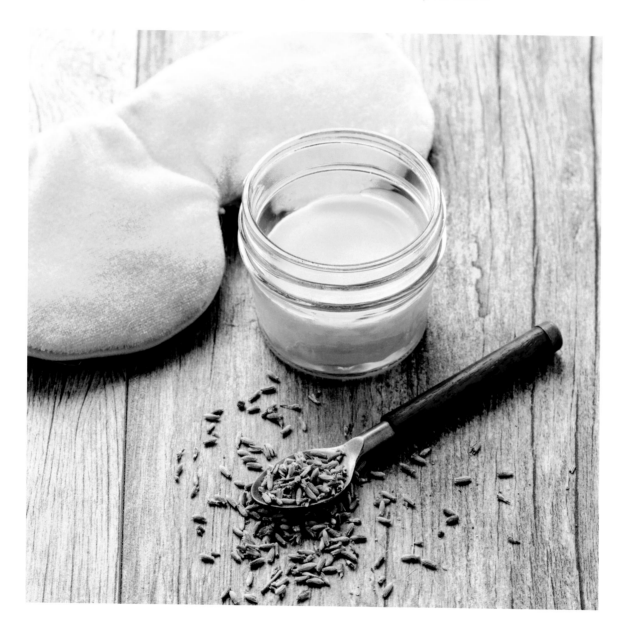

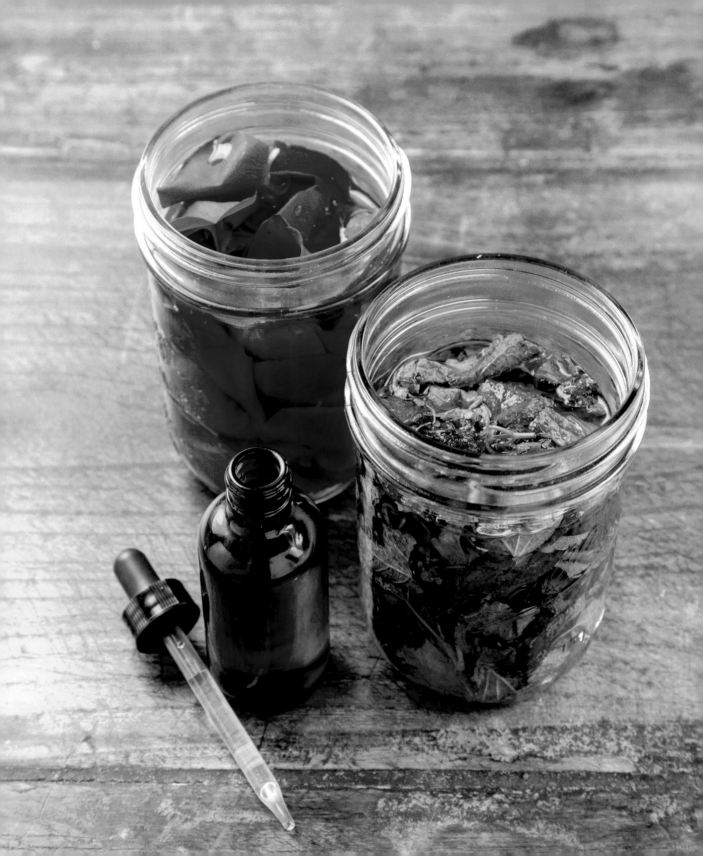

# LEMON BALM & ROSE DROPS

Several years ago, I was at one of the handmade swaps I mentioned in my Hot Honey recipe (page 72) when I found a bottle of lemon balm and rose drops that spoke to me. I added it to the other goodies I'd collected, not knowing just how important this small, unassuming bottle would become. Whenever my eldest son Huxley or I would find ourselves in moments of deep stress, panic, or anxiety, we'd have a dose of it. Made by herbalist, artist, mama, and general wise woman Adrianne Herman, this deeply calming tincture takes effect quickly, offering relief to kiddos and adults alike. This relaxed effect owes to the ability of lemon balm to increase the sensitivity of the neurotransmitter GABA, which regulates stress and sleep cycles, helping to instill a sense of calm, while rose extract has antianxiety and antidepressant properties. Additionally, both lemon balm, with its heady lemon scent, and rose, with its seductive floral aroma, induce relaxed states from their fragrances alone. I asked Adrianne if she'd be willing to share her recipe, and she graciously accepted my solicitation. Be aware that it takes nine weeks to prepare this tincture, so plan ahead. This recipe also makes a good amount of finished infusion, a quart each of lemon balm and rose, making it an ideal item to gift to friends, family, and yourself.

Yield: About 2 quarts (about 2 liters) • Frequency of use: Use in times of sudden stress or stressful events. Repeat up to four times daily, every 2–3 hours, as needed, using the dosage outlined in step 5. • Storage: Store in a cool, dark location. Use within 2 years.

## » To Prepare:

1. Fill one 8-ounce (240 ml) jar loosely with the first leaves from the lemon balm plant, and the other with rose hips. Pour vodka over the lemon balm, letting the alcohol gently flow through the empty spaces. Pour tequila over the rose hips in the same manner. Cover the jars with lids, and set them aside in a cool, dark, quiet location to infuse for three weeks. Remember to label the containers before storing. Swirl the jars gently once a week, being mindful to never turn them upside down. (According to Adrianne, this is a no-no for nerve medicines, as it agitates the plant too much, energetically speaking.)

2. At the end of three weeks, gather enough mature lemon balm leaves and rose petals to loosely fill two separate 16-ounce (480 ml) containers. Strain the first batches you infused into their

Lemon balm (early blooms,
mature leaves, stems, and
flower petals)*

Roses (hips, petals, and entire
flowers)*

3 cups (360 ml) vodka
(for the lemon balm)

3 cups (360 ml) tequila
(for the rose hips)

Two 8-ounce (240 ml) jars

Two 16-ounce (480 ml) jars

Four quart-size (1 L) jars

*These amounts will vary for each
person, as no two plants will have
leaves, stems, and flowers of equal
size. That's perfectly fine — having
exact quantities isn't necessary,
as long as you have enough plant
matter to follow the guidelines
detailed in the steps on pages
93–94. This tincture is best when
made with fresh plant matter, so
you'll want to seek out (or, better
yet, plant your own!) lemon balm
and rose plants. You'll be harvesting
from the plants across spring into
summer.*

respective jars of fresh plants. Top off the lemon balm jar
with vodka, and the rose jar with tequila. Set aside in a cool,
dark, quiet location for another three weeks, remembering to
gently swirl the jars once weekly.

3. For the third and final harvest, here are Adrianne's words:
"Roses are now ridiculous and lush, lemon balm has literally
staked claim in places you couldn't imagine, pushing up some
hue of periwinkle flowers. Get gnarly with huge leaves, flower
buds, and even some tender stem bits of the lemon balm.
Behead the huge rose and include its meaty heart."

Place these bits of lemon balm and rose into separate quart-
size (1 L) jars. As with step 2, strain and pour the second
batches over the new and final harvest, topping off the jars
with their respective alcohols. Set aside for three more weeks,
gently swirling the jars once weekly.

4. At the end of three weeks, strain the blends into new, clean,
separate quart-size (1 L) jars. When ready to combine, for
personal use or for gifting, combine the two blends in 2- or
4-ounce (60- or 120- ml) jars; each container should have a
1:3 ratio of rose to lemon balm infusion. Cap each bottle with
a dropper lid.

5. To use, administer a dropperful (about 30 drops), either
diluted in water or directly onto the tongue. You can also
add the drops to a cup of tea. Adults can repeat this dose up
to four times daily, every 2–3 hours. For children, after the
initial full dose, repeat with 3–4 drops up to four times daily,
every 2–3 hours.

# ELECTROLYTE REPLENISHER

No matter how hard you try to prevent it, someone in your house is eventually going to succumb to a stomach bug or food poisoning. When that happens, turn to this beverage. Easily made from standard kitchen ingredients, it'll help replace essential electrolytes, minerals, and nutrients lost from vomiting and diarrhea. The sea salt works to replace electrolytes, while the sweetener adds an easily assimilable form of energy. The lemon provides both flavor and cleansing properties, giving the mixture a highly palatable lemonade-like flavor. It'll be easy to persuade those who are down for the count to sip on this tart and sweet beverage.

**Yield:** About 4 cups (960 ml) • **Frequency of use:** Consume as needed throughout the day, drinking up to 8 cups (2 L) daily. • **Storage:** Store in the refrigerator, and use within 3–5 days.

## » To Prepare:

1. Place all the ingredients in a jar. Cover with a lid, and shake vigorously until fully combined. Remember to label the container.

2. Consume throughout the course of a day.

## » You Will Need:

4 cups (960 ml) cold water

Juice from 2 lemons, preferably organic*

½ teaspoon sea salt

2 tablespoons maple syrup or honey

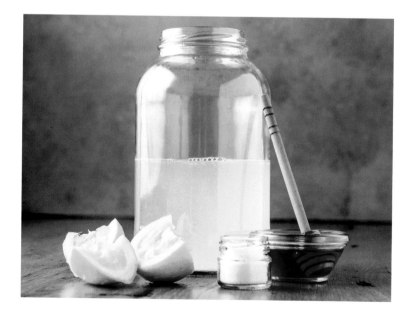

*You can swap out the lemons for limes or oranges here.*

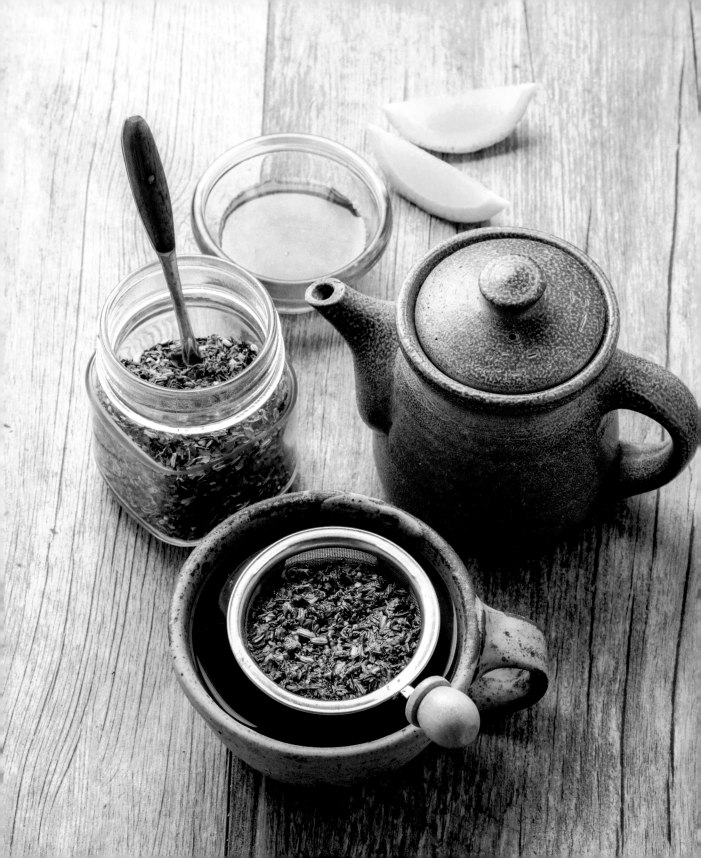

# TUMMY TEA

From my early twenties into my thirties, I had a tumultuous relationship with my digestive system. So much so, in fact, that my friends would call and inquire how I was doing and then ask how my stomach was doing, as if it were its own entity apart from my body. In an attempt to avoid taking prescription medications, I tried every natural remedy I read about or came across. It was a store-bought tea blend that finally offered the solace I sought. This is my iteration of the belly-soothing herbal concoction that brought so much relief to my distressed stomach all those years ago. I've found that it soothes stomachaches, nausea, and heartburn equally well.

Yield: ½ cup (16 g) loose tea, 4 cups (960 ml) prepared • Frequency of use: Take as needed, up to 8 prepared cups daily. • Storage: Store at room temperature out of direct sunlight. Use within 3–4 months.

## » To Prepare:

1. Place all the herbs in a mixing bowl. Stir with a spoon to combine. If not using all of the tea right away, store in an airtight container. Remember to label the container.

2. For a full teapot, place the tea blend in a ceramic or heatproof glass teapot or container. Pour 4 cups (960 ml) boiling water over the herbs. Cover with a lid and steep 15–20 minutes. For an individual cup of tea, place 2 tablespoons of the tea blend in a mug and pour 1 cup (240 ml) of boiling water over the leaves. Cover with a lid and steep 5–7 minutes. Serve as is, or with honey and lemon wedges.

## » You Will Need:

3 tablespoons dried spearmint

3 tablespoons dried peppermint

1 tablespoon fennel seeds

1 tablespoon dried tarragon

2 teaspoons dried ginger root*

Honey and lemon wedges, to serve (optional)

One 4-ounce (118 ml) airtight container

* If dried ginger root isn't available, feel free to substitute with 1 tablespoon fresh ginger, grated or cut up into matchsticks.

# HEALTHY MOUTH TOOTH POWDER

Making your own tooth powder is as easy as it is economical. It's likely that you've already got baking soda, cloves, and cinnamon in your kitchen cupboard, so you only need a few more items to get started. This powder can be used in place of toothpaste, or as a supplement to it. I like to alternate between the two every few days. Bentonite clay is known for its detoxifying properties, while calcium powder helps with whitening. Xylitol is a naturally derived sweetener that prevents bacteria from sticking to the surface of teeth; it can be found wherever alternative sweeteners are carried.

**Yield:** About ¾ cup (180 g)  •  **Frequency of use:** Use twice daily, or whenever you brush your teeth.  •  **Storage:** Store in a lidded container in a cool, dry location out of direct sunlight. Use within 3–4 months.

*Note: It's best to avoid swallowing the tooth powder, because it contains essential oil. If a small amount is swallowed, though, no need to call Poison Control. It's only larger amounts to be concerned about (for instance, your dog or baby eats nearly the entire amount of tooth powder).*

## » You Will Need:

¼ cup (65 g) bentonite clay

¼ cup (56 g) calcium powder

2 tablespoons baking soda

1½ tablespoons xylitol powder

2 teaspoons ground cloves

2 teaspoons ground cinnamon

5 drops peppermint essential oil

One 8-ounce (237 ml) glass or ceramic container

## » To Prepare:

1. Place all the ingredients except for the peppermint essential oil into a medium mixing bowl. Stir together with a wooden spoon or wooden chopstick until fully combined.

2. Drop in the peppermint essential oil. Stir until well incorporated into the dry mixture.

3. Transfer the blend to a glass or ceramic container. Remember to label the container. Secure with a lid. The mixture is shelf-stable, so it's perfectly fine to leave it out on your bathroom counter or in a medicine cabinet until needed.

4. To use, take a pinch of the powder and put it into the palm of your hand. Using your other hand, scoop up the powder with a wet toothbrush, coating all of the bristles with the powder. Brush for 2 minutes, spit out completely, and then rinse out your mouth with water (as with regular toothpaste from a tube). Follow up with flossing and Feeling Fresh Mouthwash (page 103).

5. If there are multiple members of your household, you might want to create individual batches of the powder per person, or divvy up one batch amongst the required number of jars. Small quarter-pint (120 ml) canning jars are handy for such purposes.

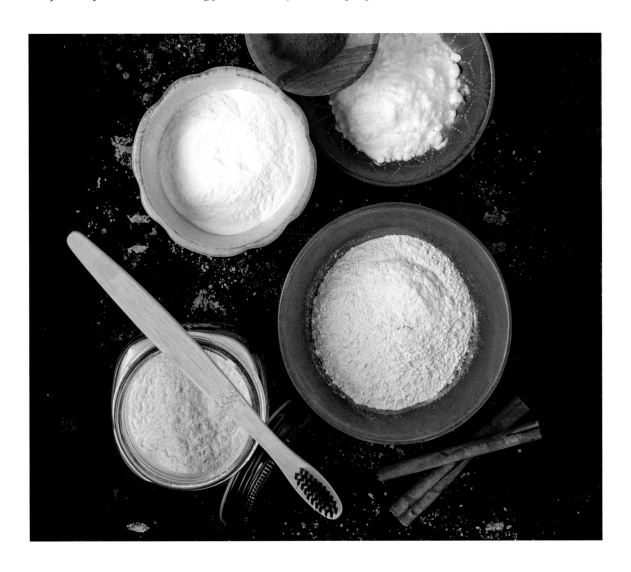

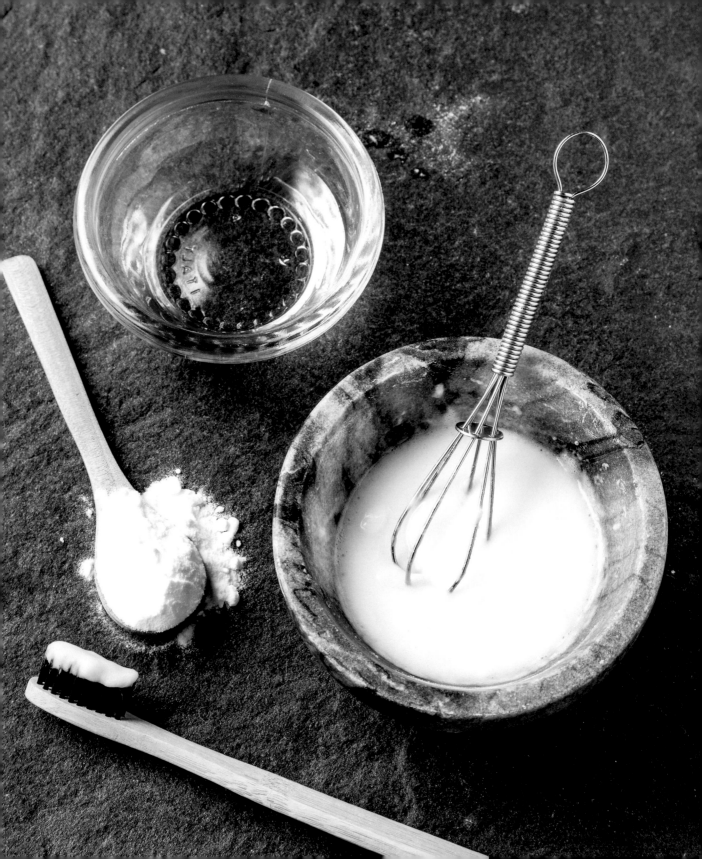

# PEARLY WHITES TOOTH WHITENER

I enjoy black tea, coffee, and red wine as much for their flavors as for their health and wellness benefits. What I don't enjoy, though, is their propensity for staining and darkening teeth. This is where this simple, natural homemade tooth whitener comes into play. Consisting of a mere two ingredients, it's incredibly cost-saving while being gently effective. Just be sure not to overdo your use of it, as using it too frequently can worsen, instead of improving, overall dental health.

Yield: 1 application • Frequency of use: Use no more than two or three times a week. Excessive use of baking soda can break down tooth enamel over time and cause tooth sensitivity. • Storage: Do not store. Use immediately.

Note: *It's best to avoid swallowing this tooth whitener, but it's not harmful if you accidentally do so.*

## » To Prepare:

1. Combine the hydrogen peroxide and baking soda in a small dish. Dip a wet toothbrush into the mixture, making sure all of it gets onto the brush, and start brushing.

2. Leave the paste in your mouth for about a minute, and then spit everything out completely.

3. Rinse your mouth out afterward with water until no hydrogen peroxide or baking soda residue remains.

## » You Will Need:

2 tablespoons hydrogen peroxide

1 tablespoon baking soda

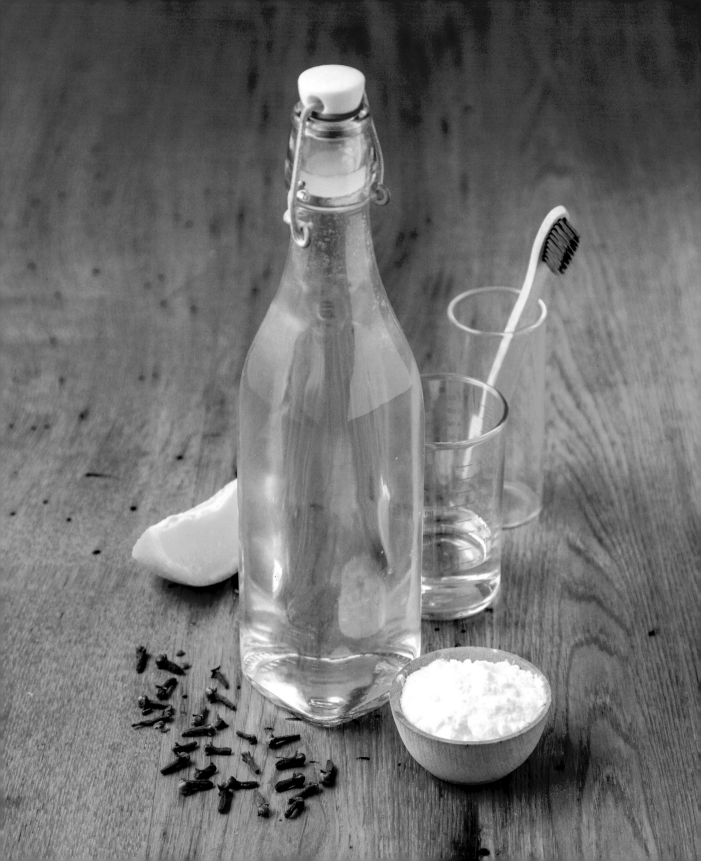

# FEELING FRESH MOUTHWASH

After brushing and flossing, a nightly rinse of mouthwash is part of my family's dental health regimen. It loosens up any remaining bits of food and keeps the entire mouth smelling fresh. Witch hazel soothes any irritated skin within the mouth and has antimicrobial and anti-inflammatory properties. Baking soda helps neutralize mouth odors and acids created by oral bacteria.

Yield: About 2 cups (480 ml) • Frequency of use: Use once or twice daily, after brushing teeth. Storage: Store in a lidded container in a cool, dry location out of direct sunlight. Aim to use the entire amount up within 2–4 weeks. Otherwise, you'll need to keep the mouthwash refrigerated.

Note: It's best to avoid swallowing this mouthwash, because it contains essential oils. If a small amount is swallowed, though, no need to call Poison Control. It's only larger amounts to be concerned about (for instance, your dog or baby eats nearly the entire amount of mouthwash).

## » To Prepare:

1. In a small mixing bowl, whisk together the carrier oil and peppermint, clove, and orange essential oils.

2. Transfer the mixture to an 8-ounce (240 ml) jar. Add the water, witch hazel, baking soda, and liquid stevia. Cover with a lid and shake vigorously until fully combined. Remember to label the container before storing.

3. When ready for use, shake entire bottle. Pour about 2 tablespoons into a cup. Tip into your mouth, swish around for 30–45 seconds, and then spit out, taking care to avoid swallowing.

## » You Will Need:

1 teaspoon carrier oil (such as jojoba, sweet almond, or grapeseed)

5 drops peppermint essential oil

3 drops clove essential oil

2 drops orange essential oil

2 cups (480 ml) distilled water

2 tablespoons witch hazel

1 teaspoon baking soda

5 drops liquid stevia

One 8-ounce (240 ml) jar

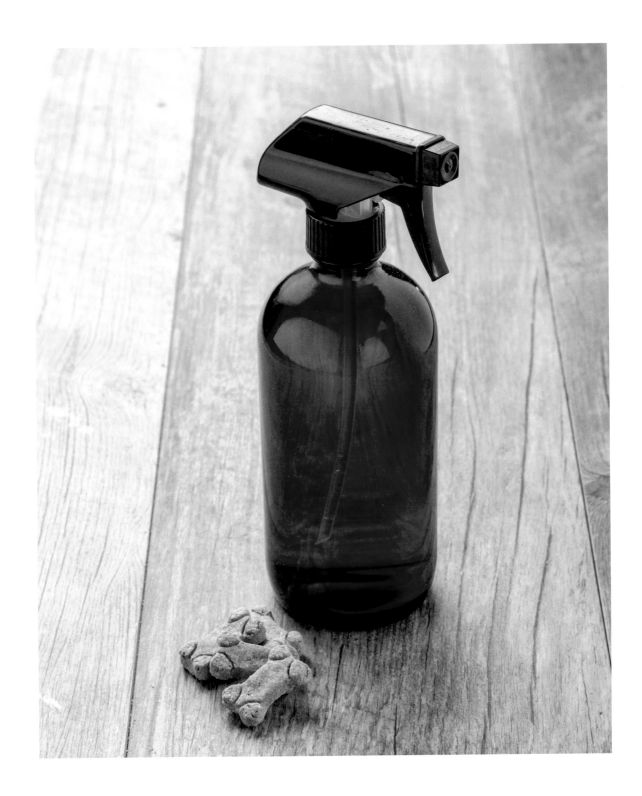

# DOGGONE ODOR ELIMINATOR

Despite our best efforts, sometimes our pets just smell like, well, animals. Our dog Dexter would most definitely prefer the fragrance of whatever dead thing he rolled around in to the fresh-from-the-groomer scent we're partial to. When you find yourself in between shampoo sessions for Fido or Fluffy, spritz a bit of this natural odor eliminator on their sleeping areas. While it won't take the place of a full washing, it helps abate the less pleasant aromas of your dogs and cats. (Don't worry, the vinegar scent dissipates quickly!)

Yield: 2 cups (480 ml) • Frequency of use: Spray on pet bedding areas, up to twice daily.
Storage: Store in a cool, dry location out of sunlight. Use within 1 year.

## » To Prepare:

1. Place the vinegar and water into a glass or plastic spray bottle. Shake vigorously to fully combine. Remember to label the bottle.

2. Spray liberally on furniture, rugs, and pet bedding whenever you need to freshen an area.

## » You Will Need:

1 cup (240 ml) white vinegar

1 cup (240 ml) distilled water

One 16-ounce (480 ml) spray bottle

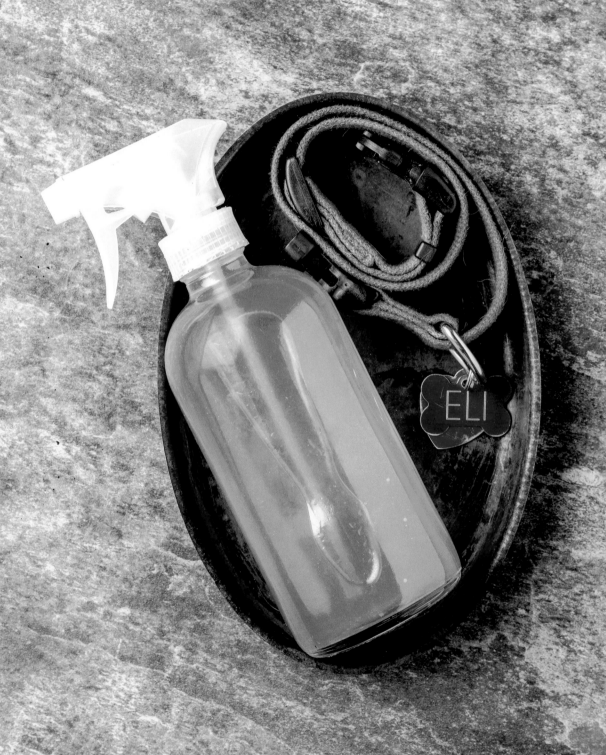

# HAPPY DAYS FLEA REPELLENT

No creature — dog, cat, or human — welcomes the bites and diseases that fleas bring. While administering flea-killing medications certainly has its advantages in terms of efficacy, doing so isn't always the best choice. Such medications are toxic to humans, posing a concern if you have little ones in the home who like to snuggle up and cuddle the home's furry friends. I take a preventative approach to flea management by spraying this naturally derived DIY repellent on my animals in flea season (typically April–October here in western North Carolina). Apple cider vinegar doesn't kill fleas; but it acts as a deterrent, since fleas don't like how it smells or tastes. Cedar essential oil is also a flea repellent thanks to its off-putting (to fleas) aroma.

Yield: 2 cups (480 ml) • Frequency of use: Begin spraying right before the start of flea season in your area. Use twice weekly, once every 3 or 4 days, all flea season long. If you live in an area that never gets cold over the winter, it's best to use this spray year-round.
Storage: Store in a cool, dry location out of sunlight. Use within 6 months.

## » To Prepare:

1. Place the vinegar, water, and cedar essential oil into a glass or plastic spray bottle. Remember to label the bottle. Shake vigorously to fully combine.

2. Spray liberally onto your pet's coat twice weekly, taking care to avoid its eyes and the entire front of its face. Use a grooming brush to distribute thoroughly and evenly.

## » You Will Need:

1 cup (240 ml) apple cider vinegar

1 cup (240 ml) distilled water

3 drops cedar essential oil

One 16-ounce (473 ml) spray bottle

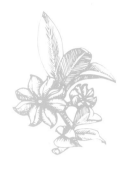

# Resources

Activated Charcoal, Arrowroot, Beeswax, Carrier Oils, Clays & Herbs

**Aura Cacia**
844-550-7200
auracacia.com

**doTERRA**
800-411-8151
doterra.com
*(Their fractioned coconut oil is a lovely carrier oil that remains liquid in all temperatures.)*

**Frontier Natural Products Co-op**
800-669-3275
frontiercoop.com

**Mountain Rose Herbs**
800-879-3337
mountainroseherbs.com

**Starwest Botanicals**
800-800-4372
starwest-botanicals.com

Calcium Powder, Citric Acid & Xylitol Powder

**Now Foods**
888-669-3663
nowfoods.com

Essential Oils

**Aura Cacia**
844-550-7200
auracacia.com

**doTERRA**
800-411-8151
doterra.com

**Floracopeia**
866-417-1149
floracopeia.com

**Simplers**
800-229-2512
simplers.com

## Natural Flavorings

**Frontier Natural Products Co-op**
800-669-3275
frontiercoop.com

**Simply Organic**
844-550-7100
simplyorganic.com

## Natural Colorings

**India Tree**
800-369-4848
indiatree.com

**Watkins**
800-928-5467
watkins1868.com

## Bottles & Jars

**Ball & Kerr**
800-240-3340
freshpreserving.com

**Weck**
815-356-8440
weckjars.com

**SKS Bottle and Packaging**
518-880-6980
sks-bottle.com

## Labels

**Avery**
800-462-8379
avery.com

**Etsy**
800-328-5933
etsy.com

## Candy Thermometers

**King Arthur Flour**
800-827-6836
kingarthurflour.com

**Oxo**
800-545-4411
oxo.com

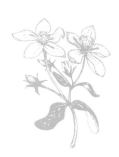

# Glossary

*Acetic Acid.* Also known as ethanoic acid, acetic acid is one of the simplest carboxylic acids. This organic compound gives vinegar its pungent aroma and characteristic sour flavor.

*Alpha Hydroxy Acids (AHAs).* A group of acids that exfoliate the outermost layers of skin, helping it become more hydrated, firmer, and smoother over time. AHAs include citric, glycolic, lactic, malic, and tartaric acids.

*Analgesic.* Any substance that can ease or eliminate pain.

*Antibacterial.* Having the ability to curtail and inhibit the growth of bacteria.

*Antimicrobial.* Having the ability to destroy or inhibit the growth of a variety of microorganisms, including bacteria, viruses, fungi, and protozoa.

*Anti-inflammatory.* Having the ability to reduce swelling and the body's inflammatory response.

*Carrier Oil.* A plant- or nut-derived oil used to dilute essential oils that might otherwise burn or harm the skin if applied directly. They typically have no fragrance of their own. Examples include jojoba, sweet almond, apricot kernel, safflower, and avocado.

*Clay.* Sourced from soil inside the earth, cosmetic clays help remove impurities from the skin, as well as absorb moisture. Clays used in this book include kaolin and bentonite.

*Collagen.* The most abundant protein in the body, making up a large part of the composition of numerous body parts, including tendons, ligaments, skin, and muscles. It provides structure to skin and strength to bones.

*Crack Stage.* The stage sugar reaches when being boiled, at which point long threads begin to form. Soft crack stage is reached around 270–290°F (132–143°C), while the hard crack stage occurs between 298° and 310°F (148° and 154°C).

*Epsom Salts.* The common name of the inorganic salt magnesium sulfate, used to soothe sore muscles, support stress reduction, reduce pain and swelling, and improve skin tone and circulation.

*Essential Oils.* A concentrated liquid containing the volatile aromatic compounds of a plant, typically obtained by steam distillation. They are called "essential" because they contain the unique essence of a plant's aroma.

*Exfoliation.* The removal of dead skin cells from the face and body by an abrasive substance or texture.

*Humectant.* A substance that retains and preserves moisture.

*Organic.* As it relates to food, those items produced or derived without the use of chemically derived fertilizers, stimulants, antibiotics, or pesticides.

*pH.* A scale, ranging from 0 to 14, used to determine acidity and alkalinity. Solutions that are more acidic have a lower pH, while more alkaline solutions have a higher pH. Neutral substances, those neither acidic nor alkaline in nature, typically have a pH of 7.

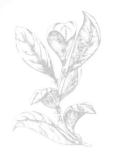

# Acknowledgments

In book writing, as in life, nothing is done solely on one's own. An invisible crew stands behind every project, every accomplishment, and every creation. *Home Apothecary* wouldn't have come to fruition were it not for a host of helping hands along the way.

Thank you to my editor, Elysia Liang, for accommodating my multiple requests at extending the deadline for delivery of my manuscript. We make our plans, and then life steps in. Heartfelt gratitude for being so gentle and understanding when life stepped in *an awful* lot in 2017 and 2018. I appreciate your flexibility and willingness to work with me more than you know. I'm also deeply grateful to the many individuals at Sterling who had a hand in bringing this book to life, including Jaime Chan, Shannon Plunkett, David Ter-Avanesyan, and Chris Bain.

Erin Adams, you were a dream photographer to work with! Sincerest appreciation for offering up your home to use as the shoot location, for keeping us both fed and properly caffeinated, and being so laid back about everything while providing professionalism behind the lens.

Deepest gratitude to Gary and Sabrina Lutes, who offered up a space in their home for me to use as a writing studio. Having that quiet place to turn to, while baby Alistair was safely at home with my husband, was a refuge beyond description.

I am eternally grateful for the teachers and wisdom keepers from whom I have had the immense fortune of learning over the years, imparting their knowledge of plants and herbs, both in person and through writings of their own. Rosemary Gladstar, Juliet Blankespoor, Luke Cannon, and Asia Suler have offered me profound wisdom, insight, and inspiration. A river of gratitude is flowing in your direction.

Thank you to my dear friend Adriana Oliviera, for both her ideas of hot honey and a milk of magnesia–based deodorant. You are always full of clever tips, hacks, and insights, and I appreciate you and your friendship deeply.

Nicole McConville was my editor for the first four books in the Homemade Living series, guiding me through *Keeping Chickens*, *Canning & Preserving*, *Home Dairy*, and *Keeping Bees* with wisdom and sage, seasoned advice. My literary career would quite literally not have launched without you. Adding to this series, with *Home Apothecary*, is a tribute to the foundation of support you provided, and I thank you from the bottom of my heart.

Finally, and always, thank you to my husband, Glenn. You don't just have my back; you're the spine running through it. You support me in silent, crucial ways. This book wouldn't have been written had you not stepped in, time after time, to watch the kids, keep me fed, and quietly cheer me on from the sidelines. Everything I do, it's because of you and your tireless support.

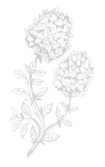

# About the Author

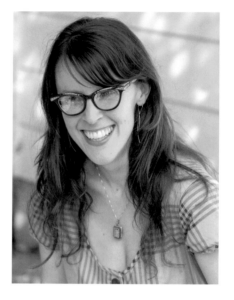

*Ashley English* holds degrees in holistic nutrition and sociology. She has worked over the years with a number of nonprofit organizations committed to social and agricultural issues, and regularly contributes to a number of international, national, and regional publications. She is the author of all four books in the Homemade Living series (*Canning & Preserving*, *Keeping Chickens*, *Keeping Bees*, and *Home Dairy*), as well as *A Year of Pies*, *Quench*, *Handmade Gatherings*, *A Year of Picnics*, *The Essential Book of Homesteading*, and *Southern from Scratch*.

Ashley lives in the mountains of western North Carolina with her husband Glenn, their two sons Huxley and Alistair, and a menagerie of animals. She chronicles her adventures in cooking, homesteading, parenting, and more at smallmeasure.com.

# Index